Evil, Te
Psychiatry

Evil, Terrorism & Psychiatry

Edited by

Donatella Marazziti
Professor of Psychiatry, University of Pisa, Italy

Stephen M. Stahl
Professor of Psychiatry, University of California at San Diego

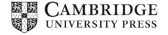

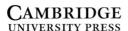

UNIVERSITY PRESS

University Printing House, Cambridge CB2 8BS, United Kingdom

One Liberty Plaza, 20th Floor, New York, NY 10006, USA

477 Williamstown Road, Port Melbourne, VIC 3207, Australia

314–321, 3rd Floor, Plot 3, Splendor Forum, Jasola District Centre, New Delhi – 110025, India

79 Anson Road, #06–04/06, Singapore 079906

Cambridge University Press is part of the University of Cambridge.

It furthers the University's mission by disseminating knowledge in the pursuit of education, learning, and research at the highest international levels of excellence.

www.cambridge.org
Information on this title: www.cambridge.org/9781108467766
DOI: 10.1017/9781108569095

© Donatella Marazziti and Stephen M. Stahl 2019

This publication is in copyright. Subject to statutory exception and to the provisions of relevant collective licensing agreements, no reproduction of any part may take place without the written permission of Cambridge University Press.

First published 2019

Printed in the United Kingdom by TJ International Ltd. Padstow Cornwall

A catalogue record for this publication is available from the British Library.

Library of Congress Cataloging-in-Publication Data
Names: Marazziti, Donatella, editor. | Stahl, Stephen M., 1951– editor.
Title: Evil, terrorism & psychiatry / edited by Donatella Marazziti, Stephen M. Stahl.
Description: Cambridge, United Kingdom ; New York, NY : Cambridge University Press, 2019. | Includes bibliographical references and index.
Identifiers: LCCN 2018043274 | ISBN 9781108467766 (pbk.)
Subjects: | MESH: Terrorism – psychology | Suicide – psychology | Violence – psychology
Classification: LCC RC454.4 | NLM WM 172.5 | DDC 616.89–dc23
LC record available at https://lccn.loc.gov/2018043274

ISBN 978-1-108-46776-6 Paperback

Cambridge University Press has no responsibility for the persistence or accuracy of URLs for external or third-party internet websites referred to in this publication and does not guarantee that any content on such websites is, or will remain, accurate or appropriate.

....

Every effort has been made in preparing this book to provide accurate and up-to-date information that is in accord with accepted standards and practice at the time of publication. Although case histories are drawn from actual cases, every effort has been made to disguise the identities of the individuals involved. Nevertheless, the authors, editors, and publishers can make no warranties that the information contained herein is totally free from error, not least because clinical standards are constantly changing through research and regulation. The authors, editors, and publishers therefore disclaim all liability for direct or consequential damages resulting from the use of material contained in this book. Readers are strongly advised to pay careful attention to information provided by the manufacturer of any drugs or equipment that they plan to use.

Contents

Contributors

Dinesh Bhugra
Institute of Psychiatry, Psychology and Neuroscience, King's College London, London, UK

Bernhard Bogerts
Salus-Institut, Magdeburg, Germany

Claudio Bonito
Università Europea di Roma, Rome, Italy

Stephanie Breitschuh
Salus-Institut, Magdeburg, Germany

Alberto Carrara
Università Europea di Roma, Rome, Italy

Marina V. Gresko
Department of Radiation Psychoneurology, National Research Center for Radiation Medicine of National Academy of Medical Sciences of Ukraine, Kyiv, Ukraine

Patrick Lemoine
Department of Psychiatry, Clinique Lyon Lumière, Lyon, France

Tatiana K. Loganovskaja
Department of Radiation Psychoneurology, National Research Center for Radiation Medicine of National Academy of Medical Sciences of Ukraine, Kyiv, Ukraine

Konstantin N. Loganovsky
Department of Radiation Psychoneurology, National Research Center for Radiation Medicine of National Academy of Medical Sciences of Ukraine, Kyiv, Ukraine

Donatella Marazziti
Dipartimento di Medicina Clinica e Sperimentale, Section of Psychiatry, University of Pisa, Pisa, and Fondazione BRF Onlus – Institute for Research in Psychiatry and Neuroscience, Lucca, Italy

Icro Maremmani
G. De Lisio Institute of Behavioural Sciences, and Santa Chiara University Hospital, Department of Specialty Medicine, University of Pisa, Pisa, Italy

Donato Marzano
Italian Navy, Italian Fleet, Rome, Italy

Anne Maria Möller-Leimkühler
Department of Psychiatry and Psychotherapy, Ludwig-Maximilians-University of Munich, Munich, Germany

Matteo Pacini
G. De Lisio Institute of Behavioural Sciences, Pisa, Italy

Armando Piccinni
Dipartimento di Medicina Clinica
e Sperimentale, Section of
Psychiatry, University of Pisa and
Fondazione BRF Onlus – Institute
for research in psychiatry and
neuroscience, Lucca, Italy

Stefano Salvatori
Departimento di Medicina Clinica e
Sperimentale, Section of Psychiatry,
University of Pisa, Italy

Maria Schöne
Salus-Institut, Magdeburg, Germany

Dorte Sestoft
Ministry of Justice, Clinic of
Forensic Psychiatry, Blegdamsvej,
Copenhagen, Denmark

Stephen M. Stahl
Department of Psychiatry,
University of California at San
Diego, San Diego, CA, USA

Guido Traversa
Università Europea di Roma, Rome,
Italy

Erich Vad
Department of International
Relations, Geschwister-Scholl-
Institute for Political Sciences,
Ludwig–Maximilians–University
of Munich, Munich, Germany

Antonello Veltri
Fondazione BRF Onlus – Institute
for research in psychiatry and
neuroscience, and Dipartimento
della Salute Mentale e Dipendenze,
Azienda USL Toscana Nord Ovest,
Pisa, Italy

Antonio Ventriglio
Department of Mental Health,
Department of Clinical and
Experimental Medicine, University
of Foggia, Foggia, Italy

Natalia A. Zdanevich
Department of Radiation
Psychoneurology, National
Research Center for Radiation
Medicine of National Academy of
Medical Sciences of Ukraine, Kyiv,
Ukraine

Foreword

No one is willingly evil, but one can become evil for a bad disposition in his body and for a training without a true education; this is hideous for everyone and happens against his will (Plato, *Timaeus*, 86e). This citation alone would suffice to show how understanding behavior has fascinated humans since ancient times.

Over the last few decades, the development of behavioral neuroscience has fostered the study of the biological correlates that subtend the mental processes involved in moral choices and social behavior. Novel brain-imaging methodologies, including positron emission tomography (PET), magnetic resonance imaging (MRI) and high-resolution electro-encephalography (EEG-mapping), have allowed scientists to adventure into the marvellous morphological and functional architecture of the human brain in an unprecedented manner. Furthermore, techniques such as transcranial magnetic stimulation (TMS) have made it possible to probe the brain by inducing temporary functional perturbations in selected cortical regions.

At the same time, the decoding of the human genome has paved the way to the study of the role of different genetic alleles in shaping personality, behavior, and vulnerability to mental disorders, as well as to understanding individual variability in response to pharmacological and even to psychotherapeutic interventions.

Neuroscience has proven to be a powerful tool to explore issues across multiple disciplines, ranging from philosophy to ethics, from economics to law, from genetics to psychiatry itself. The dialogue between social and experimental sciences has given renovated vigor to ancient questions. For instance, whether psychopathic criminals should be considered *bad* or *mad* is no longer a matter of abstract speculation, but rather has become the object of scientific investigations in which structural and functional measures in brain regions devoted to emotional processing and behavioral control are combined with evaluation of genetic factors that may affect vulnerability to aversive environmental factors during childhood. This *nature by nurture* interaction in turn may result in increased risk of expressing antisocial and impulsive behavior during adulthood. Recently, novel neuroscience advancements have entered the 2 forensic debate and the law.

In view of evidence coming from neuroscience, the question of the extent to which individuals are free and responsible for their actions has taken on renewed vigor. The issue reconnects to the medieval debate in the ethical and philosophical realm on free will versus determinism, a debate whose echo resonates in the courtroom. The capability to distinguish good from bad and to decide to act in one way or another is the foundation of the criminal justice system. Indeed, on such a foundation, retributive jurisprudence, typical of all modern societies, bases culpability and imputability.

In this perspective, *Evil, Terrorism & Psychiatry* offers an original and multidisciplinary approach to the understanding of ideological terrorism. What can neuroscience tell us about the *mind*—or rather, the *brain*—of suicide bombers? Which psychopathological factors may play a role? To what extent is religious fanaticism just a matter of molecules in the brain? Can neuroscience, psychiatry, and social sciences by working together develop effective strategies to prevent terrorism sinking deep roots within society?

Readers will find themselves viewing this issue from a new angle, no doubt from a much wider perspective than we have become accustomed to hear in the evening news.

Pietro Pietrini

Psychiatrist and neuroscientist, Director of IMT School for Advanced Studies in Lucca, Italy, and Head of MoMiLab, *Molecular Mind Laboratory*, at IMT School

Preface

Evil and good have accompanied humankind from the beginning, because they are part of human nature. Men's history (and every man's history) is characterized by a constant duel between the two opposing forces and related emotions and behaviors. When evil prevails, it may produce extreme aberrations. Unavoidably, psychiatrists and criminologists have to cope with these aberrations, as very often they are asked to provide explanations for heinous behaviors that have nothing to do with being human, except that they are perpetrated by men and also, although less often, by women (it is a real novelty of the last decades that women may become as ferocious as men). The question becomes particularly pressing in specific situations, such as in times of war (Why did the Holocaust happen? Why has there been torture?), or following genocides, murder rampages or, more recently, the terrorist attacks carried out by suicide bombers that are now perpetrated everywhere, not only in traditionally recognized unstable regions like the Middle East, but also in Western countries, at the heart of what is considered the cradle of modern civilization.

It may be useless to discuss whether evil exists or does not exist, or what its main and different philosophical conceptualizations are,[1–4] when we are casual witnesses of a terrorist attack or look at the carnage following it with a deep sense of helplessness, even while relaxing on our sofa and watching on TV the dreadful images of death and destruction that the media show with no respect to the audience.

There is nothing to say except that evil does exist and we suffer increasingly its misdeeds and consequences. More important, as psychiatrists and neuroscientists, we cannot disregard the evidence that evil is part of being human, as is good, and that both are embedded in our nature, and are probably the result of the interplay between brain mechanisms and genetic and epigenetic, familial, societal, and contextual factors.

Therefore, we cannot close our eyes in front of the brutality of evil's extreme manifestations, but, on the contrary, we should try to disentangle its mysterious roots.[5,6] Obviously, there are many intrinsic obstacles to performing studies in the field of suicide bombers, and the limitations of the available studies have been widely highlighted in the literature, but one of the paramount barriers, according to us, is due to the prejudice, reluctance, and even repulsion of some specialists to investigate evil.

Our book entitled *Evil, Terrorism & Psychiatry* aims at putting together different contributions that might be helpful in understanding the psychological and/or psychopathological processes that may transform apparently normal individuals into suicide bombers, and, in light of these, at proposing effective prevention strategies.

Our opinion is that if we want to understand evil and its radical forms we have to understand aggression and violence, and the main mechanisms regulating it.[6,7] Aggression can be defined as any behavior directed towards another individual carried out with the purpose of causing harm. It is an innate mechanism that has evolved because it may lead to some benefits or negative consequences, while promoting or impeding survival and reproduction. Violence is aggression perpetrated with the goal of doing extreme harm, including death and destruction, and perhaps may be identified and overlap with evil.

The counterpart of evil/violence is the good that might result from the entirety of the so-called socio-moral emotions encompassing empathy, sense of pity and guilt, indignation for the wrong behaviors, horror from murder, theory of mind, gratitude.[8]

Violence is probably the consequence of our innate aggression that emerges when it is no longer balanced by the moral brain, so that it becomes "radical evil" and transforms "human beings as beings superfluous," as Anna Arendt has described in a very exhaustive fashion.[9]

There are many questions arising from these considerations, and some have been addressed by this book, particularly if there are any specific personality traits, psychological characteristics, or psychopathological conditions that may favor this lack of control of violence coupled with coldness, rationality, cruelty, lack of moral sense, and, in some cases, self-celebration, leading some individuals to deliberately choose to die in order to kill innocents. Unfortunately, the available data suggest a negative answer to this major issue. Similarly, negativity is a possible impact of familial poverty, economic factors, or level of education.[10]

In any case, how can we consider "normal" those subjects, generally young, often well-educated, who become religiously radical and prefer to die while anticipating a possible reward after death? Doesn't it seem like a real cognitive distortion? Who favors this distortion? What tools are used by the charismatic leader to transform people in this way? Indoctrination? Drugs?[11]

It should also be emphasized that all societies and groups have nourished what is innate human morality and have regulated the innate aggression, while establishing a code of conduct and laws to decide what is right and what is wrong, with a primary focus on not harming others while accepting authority and respecting group rules.[12] In the terrorist's mind there is a total reversal even of this normative morality, so that killing others labeled as impure, corrupted, and enemies, according to rigid religious and group norms, is the main ethical value and not murder.

According to us, terrorism and violence in general should also be approached by a thorough understanding of the neurobiological mechanisms at the basis of human aggression and moral sense, as well as by all contextual factors that may nurture or impoverish the correct balance between the two. Recent data would indicate that early alterations of brain development, following environmental stressors or genetic liability, may impair brain circuits, pathways, and differentiation and constitute a basic "vulnerability" toward a greater risk of developing psychopathology or perhaps deviant behavior.[13] In this case, subsequent life events should act through epigenetic mechanisms modulating the stress response and emotional regulation. Of interest, both serotonin transporter-s allele carriers and sensory processing sensitivity are associated with greater sensitivity to environmental stimuli in humans.[14] Taken together, these data suggest that the prevention of terrorism requires a strong interplay between different specialties, and a careful monitoring of risk factors during childhood and adolescence supported by global changes and reshaping of political choices.

Last, but not least, as mental health professionals and neuroscientists, we should never get used to or remain indifferent to terrorism and violence, as if they were normal phenomena of our societies. On the contrary, they should be acknowledged and stigmatized on every occasion and, more importantly, investigated, starting from their basic roots, while keeping in mind that although nowadays they seem to be less powerful, their resurgence may occur in all situations characterized by personal vulnerability coupled to political/economic instability, loss of traditional values, and an individual's need for recognition. Therefore, given its multifaceted nature, the prevention of terrorism should be based on an integrated coordination of international experts targeting all possible factors involved.

References

1. Calder, T. The concept of evil. In: Zalta EN, ed. *The Stanford Encyclopedia of Philosophy*. 2016. https://plato.stanford.edu/archives/win2016/entries/concept-evil.

2. Eagleton, T. *On Evil*. New Haven, CT: Yale University Press; 2010.

3. Singer, MG. The concept of evil. *Philosophy* 2004; **79**: 185–221.

4. Knoll, JL 4th. The recurrence of an illusion: the concept of "evil" in forensic psychiatry. *J Am Acad Psychiatry Law* 2008; **36**(1): 105–111.

5. Baumeister, R. *Evil. Inside Human Violence and Cruelty*. New York, NY: Henry Holt & Co.; 1999.

6. Raine, A. *The Anatomy of Violence: The Biological Roots of Crime*. London: Allen Lane; 2013.

7. Siever, LJ. Neurobiology of aggression and violence. *Am J Psychiatry* 2008; **165**: 425–442.

8. Haidt, J. The new synthesis in moral psychology. *Science* 2007; **316**(5827): 998–1002.

9. Arendt, H. *The Origins of Totalitarianism*. San Diego, CA: A Harvest Book, Harcourt, Inc.; 1951/1985.

10. Merari, A. *Driven to Death: Psychological and Social Aspects of Suicide Terrorism*. New York, NY: Oxford University Press; 2010.

11. Zimbardo, P. *The Lucifer Effect. Understanding How Good People Turn Evil*. New York, NY: Random House; 2007.

12. Kagan, S. *Normative Ethics*. Boulder, CO: Westview Press; 1998.

13. Marazziti, D. Psychiatry and terrorism: exploring the unacceptable. *CNS Spectr*. 2016; **21**(2): 128–130.

14. Homberg, JR, Schubert, D, Asan, E, Aron, EN. Sensory processing sensitivity and serotonin gene variance: insights into mechanisms shaping environmental sensitivity. *Neurosci Biobehav Rev*. 2016; **71**: 472–483.

Chapter 1

To Die to Kill: Suicide as a Weapon. Some Historical Antecedents of Suicide Terrorism

Stefano Salvatori and Donatella Marazziti

Samson: An Example From the Bible

The story of Samson and his legendary feats are widely described in the Bible. As everybody knows, his strength was located in his long hair that should not be cut in order to preserve this unique characteristic. Unfortunately, Samson revealed his secret to Delilah, his lover, and one of her servants cut his hair while he was sleeping. In this way, he lost his strength and was made blind by the Philistines. What happened later is well known: Samson was taken to a temple and asked to rest against one of its supporting pillars, where he prayed to God to recover his strength, grasped the columns and tore them down with the famous words "Let me die with the Philistines," killing himself and all the Philistines with him.

With no doubt, Samson used his suicide as a weapon and represents one of the first examples of individuals who chose death deliberately and freely in order to kill their enemies.

An Example From Aesop's Fables

A wasp was buzzing around the head of a snake, so that it became very disturbing, while stunning it over and over again. The snake felt pain because of those awful stabs, but it could not escape from the aggressor, so that it put its head under the wheel of a carriage and died together with the wasp.[1]

This Aesop's fable describes well those individuals who choose to die together with their enemies when there is no other way to escape; in other words, they prefer to kill their enemy while losing their own life. There might be different reasons for this choice: the suicide is carried out to stop the distress, or for a cognitive distortion to be stronger than the enemies, or to provoke real harm to the enemy. At the time of the Roman Empire, it was not uncommon that slaves committed suicide in order to cause economic damage to their merciless owners. This damage was very significant to the point that Roman law regulated slaves' suicide attempts: when this event occurred, his/her value decreased significantly.

Zealots

Zealots (from the Greek word *zelotes*, meaning full of zeal, excited, ardent) were the members of a Jewish political-religious party with national-theocratic roots, born in Palestine at the end of the first century BC and lasting for about three decades. Zealots followed the norms of the Pharisonical doctrine and according to Titus Flavius Josephus (103–37? BC), a Jewish historian of Greek language: "they firmly loved freedom and only God was their king and nobody else."[2] They were nationalistic and refused to pay taxes or venerate the emperor. They played a determinant role during the insurrections against the Romans in the years 70–66 BC, although they had no real cohesion and no possibility of winning.[3] When the emperor Titus Vespasian conquered Jerusalem, they entrenched themselves in the fortress of Masada near the Dead Sea, with their commandant Eleazaro, where 960 of them committed suicide as they had no chance of overcoming or surviving their enemies. Again, Josephus wrote:

> Judah Galileans ... disregard the different kinds of death and the tortures ... In Jerusalem a new form of banditism was born, the so-called ekariots or hired killers, who killed people during the day and also in the populous market town. Under their garments they hide a little dagger (called *sica* by Romans), and killed their rivals ... They called themselves zealots, as they were "zealoters" ... Their victims were mainly the brave and the nobles, the first being them full of fear and the second because of envy: they believed their only safety was the elimination of all the important people.

Some researchers consider this movement to be one of the first examples of a social mass protest of the poor against wealthy invaders, while others cast doubt on their role as the "ancestors" of partisans. Indeed, it seems these fanatics had a great impact on the masses, offering their religious and political rules to get rid of Roman domination, but their motivations were not deep, although comprising patriotism.

The Assassins

Hasan-i-Sabbah (1034?–1124) was an eminent Persian belonging to a wealthy and influential family, a member of a branch of the Ismailian Nizaris, a dissident group of the Sciite schism, also called "the old man of the mountains" or the "prince of the mountains" by the crusaders. He used to live in the fortress of Alamut, conquered in 1091, within the mountains of Elbourz, south of the Caspian Sea, in northern Persia. Because he claimed to be the reincarnation of Ismail who had come back to earth in order to make the Muslim religion prevail, in 1090 he founded a fundamentalist Muslim sect called the Assassins.[4] This name derives from the fact that the adepts very often used hashish before their actions (in Arabic the word *hachachim* means hashish smokers). His adepts were totally submissive to him and were named the "loyal subjects" (fidawis, fidais, fedayeen, the self-sacrifice men, or the faithful friends). The old man of the mountains provided them with different drugs, and made them confused in his palace full of amenities, so that, when they were awoken, they believed they were in paradise, as is also described in Marco Polo's book *The Travels of Marco Polo*.[5,6]

Well-trained, these fanatics became cold killers for political reasons with the promise of a wonderful life after death. Generally, the murders they committed were of a political-religious nature and occurred in crowded places, at courts or sacred sites, and were followed by their killing on the spot by their victims' bodyguards. It seems they did not try either to escape, or some even to react; therefore, they killed in order to be killed without, however, committing a real suicide.[5–7] To survive was shameful and a reporter of the twelfth century reports: "When each of them decided to die in this way ... [the Boss] gave him the knife that is, so-called, consecrated."

These killers terrified the Middle East for 150 years, while destabilizing different local governments, with the aim of creating uncertainty and desta-bilization, so that the Prince might become the only ruling sovereign. (Indeed, in the Muslim world, the basis of power was based on one person: when a sultan died, his troops were scattered, and if an emir died, his country became ungovernable.) Hassan ben Sabbah chose his victims carefully, while contributing to toppling the Egyptian empire of Fatimids, the caliphate of Abassids, and the empire of Seldjuk.

To facilitate his intent, he organized supporting "cells" in different towns through corruption or threats. In order to increase confusion and suspicion, they spread lies everywhere. Very often they introduced an adept among a political, military, or religious group who, after remaining silent and loyal for several years, when ordered would commit a murder. In this way, many politicians or military officers were killed: the first was Nizam al'Musk Tusi, visir of Isfahan, then the visir Fakhr-el-Shah, the sultan Melik Saha, the Egyptian calif Abu Ali Mansur, and many others. According to some sources, the Assassins also tried to kill Edward I King of England and Saladin.[8]

When the French king Philip VI planned to start a new crusade, a German priest warned him:

> Let the Assassins be cursed and repulsed. They sell themselves, they drink human blood and kill the innocents for money, and they have no care neither of the life nor of the salvation ... As the devil they disguised themselves as an angel of the light and fake habits, language, act, clothing of different people and country ... I know a unique way to warrant the care and the safety of the king: all the servants, for every duty, important or not, must be done by persons surely, totally and clearly well known.

When Hassan ben Sabbah died, the power did not pass to any of his sons, one of whom was killed because he was suspected of conspiring against him, but to one of his more trusty adepts, Kya Buzurg-Umido. The organization continued to make killings until 1256, when the Alamut fortress was defeated by Hulagu, a Mongolian leader. In 1272 the suviving adepts, now called Ismailites, moved to Lebanon taking the name of Druses, to Iran, Syria, and to India near Bombay with the name of Khodijas.

Prince Karim Aga Khan is the 47th descendant of the Nizari family.

Some Examples in South East Asia

The presence of the first Arabian merchants in eastern Asia may date back even before Mohammed's era (570–632); however, their number increased significantly after his death. It is generally believed that they sailed from the Persian Gulf to the Indian Malabar coast, which now belongs to the states of Kerala and Karnataka, as well as to Atjah on the northern side of the island of Sumatra, and to the south of China, from where they reached Solu and Mindanao in the Philippines. The spread of the Arabian merchants was an important factor in the economies of different governments, with particular reference to the trading of fragrances, spices, wood, and Indonesian gold. In fact, since the tenth century every market of that area belonged to the Arabian population, and so Arabic became the official trading language. Their importance grew together with that of the ulamas, the Muslim doctors of religion and laws, especially when the Muslims increased to constitute 20 per cent of the local population. In 1511 when the Portuguese controlled the Strait of Malacca, there was already a powerful sultanate in Atjeh, dominating the north and south of Sumatra, and another in the Solu archipelago. Unavoidably, the Arabian trade collided with the Spanish and Portuguese colonization. In 1510 the Portuguese tried to seize Calcutta and burned down the main mosque, but then were pushed back by the local population. At that time, a commercial war began and lasted for 300 years, finishing only when the English took over the land definitively.[9]

When Spain began to conquer the Philippines in 1565, besides economic interests, there were other reasons to intervene: the general hostility against the Arabian people (the Moors), and because the fall of Granada had occurred only a few decades before. The Philippines were the main base of the Spanish people: they started fighting against their rivals with religious zeal, destroyed their harbors, ships and symbols, the mosque of Brunei and the sacred graves of the Muslims in order to lessen their importance, while at the same time beginning a partially successful evangelism by the Jesuits.[10]

Unsurprisingly, the Muslims reacted. In 1512 Alphons of Albuquerque, viceroy of the Portuguese in Calcutta, described the case of a Muslim who was considered holy because he had died while fighting against the Christians. In Malabar there occurred what is considered the first suicide attack; in Atjeh and in the Philippines this kind of struggle only began in the second half of the sixteenth century. Subsequently, thousands of Muslims died and were considered *shahids*, but they soon understood they could not resist and began to frighten the Europeans with their death. In 1592 an agent of the Society of Eastern India in Malabar wrote in his report:

> Many treacherous acts perpetrated by the Moors of Malabar frightened Christians living in the coast very much so that they seldom go out without arms . . . although the Muslims who decide to kill a Christian are a few, thay are proud to do a deserving action when they die, such as the one killing a sergeant . . . even if the most part of the Moors denies these crimes are consistent with their religion.

The quoted report reflects the point of view of a European living there, but does not highlight that "the one" was a merchant blocked by the English sergeant because he was competing with some English shipping businessmen.

Later, at the end of the sixteenth century, the Muslim Zayn alDin al Ma'bari, in his book entitled *The Gift of the Sacred Warriors with regard to some Actions of the Portuguese*, incited all Muslims to start a *jihad* against the Portuguese in order to stop their assaults against the Muslim community and the encroachment of their tradings. A holy war was considered necessary because their trades were stopped, the mosque destroyed, and there were many victims: in the future, those who would have died during this war should be venerated as a *shahids*, that is to say martyrs.

In any case, the aims of these suicide attacks are not comparable to current attacks, as they were mainly for economic reasons; political-religious reasons were added later.

From the point of view of the Muslims from Malabar their actions were simply a way to fight against the invasion of "their" lands by the Europeans, or even against the Hindu population. However, they never achieved significant success in this area, and terrorist activity persisted until the dawn of the twentieth century.

Differently from Malabar, in Atjeh the Muslims had their own government and started a *jihad* after their victory against the Dutch in a war lasting 35 years from 1873 to 1908. Just before the end of the war, *ulamas* replaced sultans. They built fortresses with many men and received money from surroundings villages to support the holy war, but they were too weak against a European army, and at the end of the war suicide attacks became the only way to fight.[11] Resistance to the colonial government was limited to the isolated killing of Europeans by the Atjenese Muslims that became a private method of *prang sabi* (to fight with the name of God). When a *kaffir* (infidel) was killed, the murderer hoped to reach paradise.[9,11] After the fall of the island of Jolo, some Muslim gangs began guerrilla warfare and others turned to what the Spanish called *juramentado*, or the man that swears, the so-called *fi sabil Allah*, that is, "to fight under the name of God." *Juramentados*, after a series of rituals and prayers, assaulted their enemies with the aim of killing as many as they could before being killed themselves. Many foreign soldiers died and there is no report of any *juramentado* surviving. Even after the Spanish government reached an agreement with the sultan, the *ulamas* continued to promote suicide actions through their *juramentados.*[10]

The Muslims of Malabar produced a lot of literature, poetries, and songs about the martyrdom of their *shahids* and on the *jihad* that were used in the twenty-first century to influence others to commit similar suicide attacks.[12] Therefore, it seems that since that time *ulamas* were the ideologists and sometimes also the political leaders and commanders, but very few are known to have committed suicide and to have choosen martyrdrom. There is more precise information about suicide terrorists of the nineteenth century in Malabar: generally, they were very young or very old, enthusiastic, simple and daring men, belonging to poorer classes and prone to the extreme sacrifice of their lives out of desperation.[13]

Some Notes on the Past Two Centuries

Throughout the centuries, terrorism has often been considered only a revolutionary phenomenon, in order to obtain freedom and rights, and as such even a positive phenomenon, as some of its aims were judged legitimate. Francois Noel Baboeuf (1760–1797) claimed: "Every ways are legitimate against oppressors" and Filippo Buonarroti (1761–1837) from Pisa wrote: "Nothing is criminal if it is used in order to get a sacred aim." Even before then, the Florentine Niccolò Macchiavelli (1469–1527) coined the famous sentence "The aim justifies the means."[14]

The first "terrorist bomb" (a barrel full of powder with some rockets tied on a rifle) was invented in Paris at the end of the eighteenth century and was used in 1800 by conspirators who wanted to kill Napoleon, with no success.

In 1848, when some revolutionary insurrections occurred, Karl Heinzen (1809–1880), a German radical democratic, in his book *Der Mord* (*The Assassin*) produced the thesis that a murder might be politically legal if perpetrated against a dictator. The principles of "propaganda through the action" are mentioned to justify the unsuccessful mission of Carlo Pisacane in Campania, a southern Italian region in 1857. This concept was also expressed by the Italian anarchic Enrico Malatesta (1853–1932) and Carlo Cafiero (1846–1892), who created a manifesto about it, although the former was hostile to terrorism.

The first modern work on terrorism can be considered Nachaev's (1872) book entitled *The Revolutionary Foundamental Tenets*, where it is written:

The revolutionary [terrorist] knows only one science, the science of the distruction. For this reason, and only for this reason, he will study mechanics, chemistry, and maybe medicine. During the day and the night he will study people's sociology, their peculiarities and the entire phenomena of the today's social order. The matter is always the same: the destruction of this dirty world.

According to some Russian sociologists, the terrorism was not only effective, but humanitarian. In order to get a better world, only a few had to die, favoring the community.

Herein, we list some examples of modern terrorist activities that were never suicide. From 1878 to 1913 the Narodnaya Volya (the will of the people) and the party of the Fighting Organization of the Revolutionary Socialists in Russia; the anarchic terrorism at the end of 1800 in Europe and particularly in France; the Irish Republican Army (IRA) starting in 1922; the Irgun Zwai Leumi in Palestine from 1937 to 1947 that chose individualistic terrorism; Mau-Mau in Kenya from 1952 to 1956; The National Liberation Front in Algeria from 1954 to 1962; the EOKA in Cyprus from 1957; the Islamic Jama'at El in Egypt; the Jaish Mohambut in India; the Abn Sayyaf in the Philippines; Muslim terrorism in Kashmir; the OLP in Palestine from 1968 to present; the ETA in Spain until October 2011; the Red Army Faction and the Movement of June 2 in Germany until 1968; Tupamaros in Uruguay; the Red Brigades (Brigate Rosse) in Italy between 1970 and 1987.

Only the members of the Narodnaya Volya accepted to die on the spot after an attempt with one hand granade, or when they were convicted to death after a trial: they exploited the sentence in order to further accuse the political system and to convince many observers to believe their death was not more important than their desire to kill.[14]

A Peculiar Japanese Example: the Kamikazes

Kublai Khan (1215?–1295), nephew of Genghis Khan, conquered China, became an emperor and founded the Yuan dynasty. He welcomed Marco Polo in Cambaluc, today's Peking. In 1274 he decided to conquer Japan and sailed from the Hakaka Bay towards the Japanese archipelago, but an unpredicted typhoon obliged the devastated fleet to turn back.

After seven years he tried again and landed in Kyushu Island, where he met unforeseen resistance from the local people. When his fleet composed of 4,000 ships began the decisive battle, the sun stopped shining and a huge cloud appeared in the sky, completely obscuring the daylight, even though it was only late afternoon. A violent typhoon appeared on the horizon moving toward the Mongolian fleet, the sea surged and destroyed the ships, which sank with no pity, as if unknown forces had been allied with the Japanese people to defeat their enemies.[15] Therefore, the so-called *shimpu* or *kamikaze* (*kami*: divine; *kaze*: wind), the wind of the gods, saved Japan from the Mongolian assaults, so that in subsequent centuries nobody attempted to replicate the attack. Although the word *kamikaze* entered the chronicles and the history, it is unclear when and who coined this term. A common notion is that it was coined by soldiers born in USA from Japanese-American parents who fought in the Pacific Ocean in the US Navy, but this version has never been verified. Nowadays, this word is not adopted by the Japanese press, which defines suicide terrorists with the term *jibaku tero* (auto-exploding terrorist).

In the Pacific Ocean the activities of this special corps began officially on October 25, 1944, when the course of the war in Japan was already compromised. Before this date, during the battle of Bougainville in New Guinea, Japanese soldiers threw themselves loaded with explosives against the enemy tanks, a technique called *nikudan* (bullet men). However, the results of the *nikudan* were not positive, as the Americans continued to make progress. Other scattered cases of desperate action had already occurred in the previous months. For example, in September of the same year, when some Japanese planes were shot down during an attempted suicide attack against an American carrier around the Negro Islands, or when an officer of a Japanese fighter plane successfully collided with a B-17 bomber.[16] This tactic was named *tai-atari* or clash between two corps, and led on October 21 to severe damage to the Australian flagship *Australia* by an unidentified Japanese pilot. Vice-Admiral Takijiro Onishi, a man with great charisma, proposed and obtained approval to organize a special corps, against the advice of other reliable members of the high command. It seems that even Emperor Hirohito was not convinced to continue the war, while officially adopting that kind of last-hope solution, probably without approving it. However, in view of the unfavorable state of the military operations, Onishi did not see any other way to reverse the outcome of the operations than to delay the unavoidable defeat. Unfortunately, since the Battle of Midway, American planes had conquered the sky while the Japanese airforce was decimated, and the chance of a pilot returning from a mission was unusual, which the pilot knew. "My plane shall crash to an enemy's aircraft carrier . . . and it will become a mass of metal . . . My enemies, who will die because of my attack, will also become a part of it. My plane and an enemy carrier . . . me and my enemy . . . we shall melt all together."[16] Again, "Maybe you do not understand why I am going to die . . . You and me belong to different times and then we think in different way."[17] These few lines are perfect examples of the feelings of the young pilots, generally university students between 20 and 25 years of age who became "kamikazes." Why did they accept the moral constraint to sacrifice themselves? Existing evidence would suggest that the main reason was the adherence to moral and higher order and duty. One detail is non-negligible: they were fighting in a declared war; this was a sufficient reason to kill their enemies and defend themselves and their country.

The tactic of these pilots was peculiar. Their first aim was to frighten the enemy with the noises of their famous Zero fighters, which contained 250 kg of explosives and 800 kg of bombs, inducing fear and psychological distress, and then to do real damage to the ships. A special target of their attacks was the flight decks of the American aircraft carriers, which were made of wood. Another important target to hit was the lift, an unlikely outcome because the Japanese pilots underwent only a short training of a few weeks that, unfortunately, did not include landing.[18] When the target was a troopship, a cargo ship, another ship or a convoy, the exact aim was to damage the steering instruments and then the bridge. The best result was obviously the sinking of the ship.[18,19]

After the first successful attacks, the Japanese started to build planes that were more suitable for kamikaze activity: they utilized engines that could not fly for too long and had a wooden structure; the undercarriage was neither retractile nor steady: it had to be unfastened after take-off in order to be retrieved and reused. In spite of the visualization by radars, interception and massive anti-aircraft fire, 14 per cent of the kamikaze attacks crashed on a ship, and about 8.5 per cent caused severe damage. The most important role of the kamikazes was during the last two big battles: Iwo Jima (February 1945) and Okinawa (April 1945).[20]

At the end of the war, there was a large, controversial debate among the Japanese public regarding this special corps: the main criticism being that it seemed absurd to oblige so many young men to sacrifice themselves only to prolong the agony of defeat and hide military mistakes. In his book *The End of a War*, Admiral Suzuki wrote: "The essence of the special corps elicits a religious admiration, but it symbolizes the result af the Japanese defeat".[21] Again, the US Navy commissioned a report about Japanese national spirit from the anthropologist Ruth Benedict. In her book *The Chrysanthemum and the Sword: Patterns of Japanese Culture*, she highlighted that in Japan spirituality is superior to materialism, and how much religiosity can characterize both individuals and the whole nation's sum of values and life. In Japan during the 1930s, Shintoism, the main Japanese religion, based on the values and the cult of the ancestors, shifted towards the values of the *bushido*, a set of codes and ideals inspiring the samurai's life, so that everyone's life identified with that of all the country. The *bushido* considered death as a privileged feature to join the *kami*, the spirits of the national heroes. The military ruling class introduced this principle to modify mass psychology to the point that there were many suicides among the armed forces and civilians, even when hostilities were over.[22]

The role of kamikazes has also been highly debated outside of Japan. One conclusion is that if they delayed the end of war in the Pacific Ocean, they might be one of the factors that forced the USA to use the atomic bomb in Japan. In any case, kamikazes fought neither for revenge, nor hate or fanaticism, but because their sacrifice was considered useful to their country and the emperor. Their shout *Banzai*, which means "10,000 years of life to the emperor," underlines how their life could be lost in front of the well-being of their country.[19,20] In one *haiku* (poetry), Captain Seki Yu Kio wrote: "Fall my followers / as cherry blossom / as I shall fall in a short / at the duty of my country." Again, a famous song about a kamikaze says: "If I go into the sea, my body shall come back driven by the waves / If my duty bring me on the mountains / a carpet of grass will be my blanket / To save the emperor / I shall die in peace inside my home." In one letter, a kamikaze wrote to his parents: "I am disgusted, while thinking of the tricks that innocent citizens are victims by some of our devious politicians. I accept to receive orders from the high commanders and also from the politicians because I believe in the state. The Japanese way of life is nice and I am proud of it, as of its history and mythology reporting purity . . . it is an honour to give my life in exchanging of so fine and high values."[23]

Obviously kamikaze were not terrorists, although they used suicide as a weapon.

Conclusions

In this chapter, some possible antecedents of terrorism have been reviewed and presented. It is evident that possible similarities with modern expressions of suicide terrorism are weak or non-existent. The motivations of the past examples were generally political or economic, or they represented extreme self-sacrifice for the benefit of the whole nation, such as in the case of Japanese kamikazes, or showed the birth of a national spirit, typical of some European countries of the mid-nineteenth century. In some cases, public murders were apparently driven by religious values (Palestinian Zealots, or Muslim merchants in South East Asia). Again, it was not unusual that religion had been used to mark the difference and manipulate adepts, for increasing personal power, like the old man of the mountains used to do, or by Asian ulamas to fight against invaders to reaffirm the existence of the Muslim world and heritage.

This idealistic zeal is totally lacking in modern suicide bombers. Although affirming to belong to the Muslim religion and to fight a holy war against the corrupted Western way of life, it seems that there are no other aims than those to provoke and increase terror, while killing thousands of innocents through their own deaths. As such, they represent a totally new phenomenon that requires novel and specific instruments of investigation.

Disclosures

The authors do not have any disclosures, and the authors do not have any affiliation with or financial interest in any organization that might pose a conflict of interest.

References

1. Esopo. *Favole*. Milano: Feltrinelli; 2014.

2. Josephus. *Antiquities Book XVIII*.

3. Sorek, S. *The Jews Against Rome: War in Palestine AD 66–73*. London: Bloomsbury; 2008.

4. Lockhart, L. *Hasan-i-Sabbah and the Assassins*. London: University of London; 1930.

5. Lewis, B. *Origins of Ismailism*. Cambridge: Cambridge University Press; 1940.

6. Hodgson, MGS. *The Order of Assassins*. The Hague: Mouton; 1955.

7. Poonawala, IK. *Biobibliography of Ismāʻīlī Literature*. Malibu, CA: UCLA, von Grunebaum Center for Near Eastern Studies/Undena Publications; 1977.

8. Lewis, B. *The Assassins: A Radical Sect in Islam*. Oxford: Oxford University Press; 1967.

9. Siegel, J. *Shadow and Sound. The Historical Thought of a Sumatran People*. Chicago, IL: University of Chicago Press; 1978.

10. Majul, CA. *Muslims in the Philippines*. Manila: The University of the Philippines Press; 1999.

11. Siegel, JT. *The Rope of God*. Ann Arbor, MI: University of Michigan Press; 2000.

12. Fawcett, F. War songs of the Mappilas of Malabar. *Indian Antiquary*. 1901; **30** (Nov–Dec): 499–508, 528–537.

13. Ileto, RC. *Magindanao, 1860–1888: The Career of Dato Utto of Buayan*. Manila: Anvil Vintage; 1971.

14. Della Porta, D. Life histories analysis of social movement activists. In: Diani M, Eyerman R, eds. *Studying Collective Action*. New York, NY: Sage; 1992: 168–193.

15. Arena, LV. *Samurai*. Milano: Mondadori; 2002.

16. Tolland, J. *The Rising Sun: The Decline and Fall of the Japanese Empire*. New York, NY: Random House; 1970.

17. Natsume, S, Kokoro, B. *Il cuore delle cose*. Vicenza: Neri Pozza; 2001.

18. Scherer, K. *Kamikaze: Todesbefehl fuer Japans jugend: Ueberlebende berichten*. Muenchen: Judicum Verlag; 2001.

19. Hoyt, EP. *The Kamikazes*. New York, NY: Arbor House; 1983.

20. Inoguchi, R, Nakajima, T, Pineau, R. *Vento divino. Lavera storia dei kamikaze*. Milano: Longanesi; 1953.

21. Suzuki, DT. *Selected Works of DT Suzuki*. Oakland, CA: University of California Press; 2014.

22. Benedict, R. *The Chrysanthemum and the Sword: Patterns of Japanese Culture*. New York, NY: Houghton Miffin; 1946.

23. Morris, I. *La nobiltà della sconfitta*. Modena: Guanda; 1983.

The Philosophy of Hate and Anger

Chapter 2

Claudio Bonito and Guido Traversa

Anger and Hate from a Philosophical Perspective

At first glance, it may appear that these elements belong to two different dimensions: on one side there is philosophy, identified as the correct use of rationality, which implies the ability to follow the "veining" path of reality. Plato associated this concept to the ability, possessed by philosophers, to understand relationships between genres. On the opposite side, there is anger, hate, resentment, and violence: these categories, indeed, do not seem to be interpreted on the basis of the philosophical categories.

Violence is generally considered the direct consequence of hate and anger and it seems to be constantly embedded in human nature. Several authors reached this same conclusion in times far away from neuroscience's findings; Darwin's hypothesis of the existence of an instrument with selective purposes, and, later on, Lorenz's reference to violence as a constant behavior belonging to the animal kingdom, including humans.

Philosophy seems to take a step back from all of this. It appears almost as if it does not recognize the phenomenon by choosing to maintain it outside its domains. The same attitude was present among Plato's commenters. Their evaluations could be carried out in an optimal way only if they were raised "far" from anger and violence. It is almost as if their intent was to avoid contamination and the loss of pureness in thoughts, which represents the highest capacity of evaluation.

One could say that even biblical epics were initiated by a violent act: condemnation of humanity to an earthly and strenuous existence. The background of our story is the murder of Abel by Cain.

Greek tragedians almost absolutized anger and hate when composing and presenting the series of violent and cruel facts making up the primordial myths of creation. As long as we know, those myths were later assimilated by the western Roman Empire until its decadence.

In the Middle Ages, the concept of Theodicy comprised the attempt of justifying from a theological point of view the existing part of evil that hosts hate and violence. Today, theologies, philosophies, and religions are still ashamed of its existence and its aporias.

In fourteenth-century Europe, Meister Eckhart used to preach about the concept of detachment, while passing on the image of a wise man dipped in a serene and contemplative indifference. The German mystic acquired this idea from ancient philosophical schools, and its features can be traced in the first form of stoicism, under different designations such as *apàtheia* or *ataraxia* (apathy, ataraxy, imperturbability). These concepts will be found once again in the Christian mindset, which comprises the "Incarnated Logos" and engages against anger and hate, in the doctrinal war that will place wrath among the "seven sins." On the path to absolutism, this war's features will gradually give birth to the fundamental conflict between good and evil.

As hate, anger, and violence express irrationality, the philosopher ought to observe them from a distance, in the same way a construction worker must check the progress of his building by looking at it from far away if he wishes to grasp a view of the whole.

As sons and daughters of hate, we have been condemned to live with it since the beginning of our time. We are always close to giving in to this feeling and there is not much we can do about it, except learn to use those tools that we have been given by Reason. *Sapere Aude!* In Kant's critique, it is reason itself, though, that was placed on the witness stand and left to the doors of modernity, wearing enlightenment's guise of "progress" with the objective of helping man to escape from his state of minority.

These same concepts were later used by Nietzsche's nihilist theories. These theories were securely placed on the other side of good and evil, and a glimmer of hope for the birth/rebirth of a better humanity, as a consequence of the death of God.

Similar to myths, religions often expect and demand the dangerous association to violence, anger, and hate. They even place these feelings as distinguishing and founding elements. This is the case of Christianity, a perfect example of the concept exaggerated to the point that, in the apotheosis of a rabid and violent act, violence is unleashed against the incarnated son of God himself.

As already noted, most of the religions belonging to the Ancient Near East and the so-called Abrahamic religions originate from an act of rage and violence. Not to mention the polytheisms of the Classic era, based essentially on enraged and choleric relationships between several members of the Pantheon, which portrayed the gods in a constant state of conflict one with each other.

By juxtaposing it to religion, though, we get a glimpse of something different regarding the essence of hate. Nowadays, we witness the creation of parallel pathways between violence and religions almost on a daily basis, and realise how they can turn out to be dramatically contiguous.

After September 11, 2001, world populations witnessed how lethal and dangerous this combination can be, in a historical time where world peace is threatened by what can be considered the most degraded product of rage and hate. The matrix of terrorism has today revealed its essential religious nature and this alone should be enough to impair our own rationality.

Terrorism itself has changed tune, taking on unedited modalities and making use of a weapon that openly challenges our capacity to think rationally: the human body. The human body, indeed, has become an actual "unconventional weapon," a tool used to inflict death and pain. One could bitterly hypothesize a sort of post-modern era of terrorism. Today, it imitates contemporary anthropology, leading to an abuse of the body for its malleability and adjustable properties and intensifying the concept by using it to bring pain, death, and desperation. This is how the violence of a rabid act transforms into a moment of glory, becoming martyrdom. Then, hate borders on celebration. As a consequence, those concepts, intrinsic in and approximated to rage, hate, and violence, urgently need a philosophical reinterpretation.

Our opinion is that a philosophical observatory of international experts should be created in order to approach and possibly understand modern terrorism. This observatory should indicate new ways to intervene in our current social reality to guide its evolution away from submerging man himself, by using new perspectives, while processing categories of thought that have been verified in the past.

The Spectator in Front of Hate in the Context of Television Communication: From Film to Image. Towards a Philosophy of Perception

In the Editorial of February 25, 2015, the Director of the Italian RaiNews 24, one of the main Italian public TV channels, Monica Maggioni, stated that videos belonging to the Isis propaganda would no longer be broadcast. She declared that she no longer intended to be the "sounding board" to their ideology and added that, from that moment on, she would publish only photographs or photograms.

In Sousse, in the gulf of Hammamet, on June 26, 2015, 38 people were killed during a terrorist attack on the beaches of two resorts. For days, a particular image was shown all over the world, that of one of the terrorists before being killed by the security force.

At first glance, the photograph seems to depict a tall young man with long hair, carrying something similar to a shotgun in his right arm. His head is slumped to the left, slightly leaning forward. The boy is walking at a slow pace on the waterside, with a dozen people behind. They are all men and they look as though they are acting normally. They could be playing. On the sand, to the left, there are some common sea rafts for kids. In the background there is the modern structure of the resort.

Due to its understandable simplicity, this image causes no astonishment among those who have not heard the "news" related to this visual document. The Kalashnikov looks like a speargun; the vacillating pace of the young man could induce an empathic sense of indifferent tiredness; the people and the young crowd behind the boy could be taken from a Pasolini street movie; the whale and the rubber rafts, left to dry on the beach, are turned towards the path where the young man is walking on the shore. His pace does not seem aggressive, as if he has nothing to do with war. He simply looks tired under the sun, high in the sky; who knows how many, looking at this picture, have felt some kind of overwhelming maternal instinct to alleviate the fatigue of that boy during his solemn and tired gait! This empathy, however, disappears as soon as one becomes aware of the terrible reality behind the photo.

We should ask ourselves if the feeling of empathy disappears completely and if it first transforms itself into indignation towards the attack, and then into pity towards the victims. However, what if that feeling does not completely fade but is led, by pain and surprise, to condemning terrorism; in this case, where does it go?

Using familiar terminology in a philosophical era, we feel that a conscious switch from "opinion" (*Meinung*) to "knowledge" (*Erkntniss*) is needed. One thing should be clear: the objective of this discussion is not to glorify the role played by videos to the detriment of that of fixed images: the passage from the opinion to the ethical judgment is possible with both forms of visual communication, whether it is in motion or still; a flux of connected images, though, places each photogram in a frame and helps the elaboration of the judgment; the singular image, instead, requires further information. This is a good thing because it can stimulate a form of judgment that gives importance to the singularity, whether it's symbolic or not, of what is seen as "motionless."

Therefore, it is necessary that one is ready to give out and, above all, to receive news in order to understand their true meaning and predict potential evolution. This attitude, which can be labeled as "foresightful reception," is too often absent in the spectators who, for this reason, risk losing the fundamental ethical position in the present and in history belonging to them. Opinions need foresight, acumen: to be transformed into knowledge and judgment, they must not be abandoned.

We must never give up keeping this perspective, for the simple reason that we put it into practice unconsciously every day: the perspective of a spectator. If we maintain this point of view and the appropriate foresight, we could catch certain "propensities" of the present time, even by "simply" watching the news. These "propensities," intended as physical forces which belong to the dimension of social and political history—and not only as simple possibilities—are incongruent to Gramsci's "indifference" and highlight real actions that must be taken following the "logic" of the historical present.

Viewing images after a philosophical education, which then turns into a civic education, can help pick up and distinguish possibilities for hate and violence, even before those for war or peace.

Disclosures

The authors do not have any disclosures, and the authors do not have any affiliation with or financial interest in any organization that might pose a conflict of interest

References

1. Platone. *Fedro* 265e. In: *Platone, tutti gli scritti,* a cura di Giovanni Reale. Milano: Rusconi; 1991.

2. McGinn, B, ed. *Meister Eckhart: Teacher and Preacher.* Toronto: Paulist Press; 1968: 152.

3. Laerzio, D. *Vite e dottrine dei più celebri filosofi.* Milano: A cura di Giovanni Reale, Bompiani; 2006.

4. Orazio. Epistole (I, 2, 40), trans. Rita Cuccioli Melloni. Milano: Rusconi Libri; 2016.

Identity, Alienation, and Violent Radicalization

Antonio Ventriglio and Dinesh Bhugra

Introduction

Identity as an individual or as part of a culture or community lies at the core of who we are and more importantly how we see others seeing us. As migrants or new arrivals in a culture or even within the same culture an individual develops identity in response to how they are brought up—what their world view is—and how they individuate and begin to see themselves. Furthermore, the degree of comfort and acceptance within the society and culture allows them to develop and nurture a sense of belonging and purpose and the concept of the self. Although it has been argued that concepts of individual self may vary across cultures, the degree of comfort and belonging to a group or community remains paramount and drives the healthy individual to acculturate. Alienation can contribute to poor acculturation and consequent violent radicalization as a consequence of the search for identity and belonging, and we present herein a new model linking cultural identity and violent radicalization.

Acculturation and Identity

Marks and Pick argue that keeping a focus on apparent pathologies of particular individuals may distract us from the underlying social and political circumstances alienating whole communities or large populations.[1] Therefore, under the circumstances, it is important to understand family and group acculturations and alienation. Cultural and resulting psychological adjustment and the following changes are consequent to direct or indirect contacts between two cultural groups and their individual members (Redfield et al. 1936).[2] Berry suggests that the issue of one's cultural identity depends on intercultural contacts, and cultural identity is a sense of attachment or commitment to a cultural group;[3] cultural identity and acculturation are both a cultural and a psychological phenomenon in contrast with the proposal by Graves[4] that acculturation is simply psychological. Berry defines processes of acculturation and strategies depending upon distinction between one's own cultural group and those towards the other groups.[3,5–7] In addition, he underlines that at an individual level both the behavioral changes and acculturative stresses may function at a level where people try to accept some if not all of the cultural factors of the majority/dominant or new culture.

Berry and Kim argue that acculturative stress is very common and affects psychological, somatic, and social aspects of individual functioning and, in return, it is influenced by gender, age, educational status, and cognitive styles.[8] The process of acculturation was initially conceptualized as a group process, so it is important to recognize that both individual and group levels of acculturation must be carefully recognized and studied if one is to understand the processes of violent radicalization. Alienation from the larger society or the group is bound to affect integration, and can be seen as the opposite of a sense of belonging. Alienation is an individual's feeling of unease or discomfort reflecting their exclusion or self-exclusion from social and cultural participation.[9] Seen as an expression of non-belonging, alienation creates a sense of uneasy awareness or unwelcome contrast with others. It may be restricted to a small number of focused situations, such as participative activities in certain settings, or may be a sporadic feeling arising from specific events and encounters involving one or more situations. Alternatively, it may be a continuous and/or intense feeling perpetuated by the individual's self-perception, and how he/she considers others seeing him/her, which may be a correct or exaggerated perception; thereby, depending upon other factors may create a sense of alienation. In addition, perceptions related to aspiration and achievement and socio-cultural location of the individuals may well play a role in creating this feeling.

It is entirely possible that factors which are similar or very close between the two cultures may enable and support acculturation such as diet, language, and so on, and reduce the sense of alienation, whereas differences such as religion, its practice and values may well create difficulties in adjustment by increasing a sense of isolation and alienation. Therefore, a sense of non-belonging can be real or perceived, and the perception of non-belonging may be caused by interactions with society, as society may be not welcoming because of an individual's religion, gender, sexual orientation, or other variables. It is worth recognizing that alienation may be caused by a number of factors, but also as Hajda points out by rejection by the peer group on the basis of specific encounters and events which may involve a small group of individuals, but take on major importance in the mind of the vulnerable person.[9] The sense of alienation may emerge as a result of continual chronic difficulties or sudden responses, but needs to be seen and recognized in conjunction with a sense of integration. Hajda outlines this relationship between alienation and integration and argues that the degree of alienation will be influenced by a number of factors.[9] These include the number of qualitatively different collectivities (groups) an individual belongs to and the number of subcultures they participate in (and feel accepted). The sense of belonging is important in playing a major role in one's identity and cultural and psychological acculturation. The tension between different subgroups or subcultures may affect the individual, thereby contributing to a sense of non-belonging. The support of the people important to the individual can influence this sense of belonging/non-belonging. It is unavoidable that the degree and strength of attachment to these groups will affect a sense of belonging/non-belonging. The extent to which being a member of these groups is recognized as being part of the larger societal group can reflect the values of the individual and the group, creating tension leading to alienation.

Depending on personality traits and characteristics, it is likely that this sense of primary non-belonging will be turned into belonging to a gang or subgroup with its own cultural nuances and taboos. Therefore, these individuals may experience a high degree of alienation with dissatisfaction, withdrawal or apathy, and belonging to a cult—be it religious or political—gives them a sense of purpose. Hajda raises an interesting point in that those who belong to a collectivity or a cultural subgroup may well have a sense of belonging or commitment to different sets of values, norms, and beliefs that may also be compartmentalized.[9] Others linked alienation with apathy,[10] authoritarianism,[11] political apathy,[12] or political hyperactivity,[13] prejudice,[11] and powerlessness.[14] The feelings of powerlessness may lead to feelings of helplessness and subsequent depression and suicide.[15] Marks and Pick propose that many features of the markers of a terrorist mindset can apply to most of us depending upon a number of factors.[1] They observe that of the 22 points used in a checklist for the Prevent program, which is a key part of the British government's anti-terror strategy, some of the criteria for "grooming" are too lax. They give examples of propensity for excitement and adventure, feelings of threats and insecurity, a sense of anger, and a wish for status. All of these can be applied in multiple situations. There is no doubt that many individuals who commit these acts experienced major childhood traumas. Marks and Pick suggest that indoctrination processes are often complex and are influenced by hidden persuaders.[1] There is every likelihood that the intensity of anxiey experienced by vulnerable individuals and their fantasies and projections may play a crucial role. There have been suggestions that malignant narcissism[16] and religious fervor may contribute to radicalization.

Anomie and Radicalization

The anomie of Durkheim has been redefined as normlessness which means that the individual has a sense of painful unease or anxiety, feelings of rejection or separation from the society or the group standards, and feelings of pointlessness that no certain goals exist.[17] Olsen challenges this assumption, arguing that the translation of anomie is not simply about normlessness but is more than that.[18] His argument is that Durkheim described two types of anomie. The first is inadequate procedural rules to regulate complementary relationship among the specialized and interdependent parts of a complex social system. The second described in his book on suicide is inadequate moral norms of social control. Suicides increase during times of industrial and financial crises; however, the reason for increased suicide is not poverty, but rather with "crises of prosperity" (periods of economic growth and prosperity) that lead to increased rate of suicide. Such crises are related to disturbances of the collective order. Every disturbance of equilibrium, even though it may involve greater comfort and a rise in the general pace of life, provides an impulse to voluntary death. For violent radicalization it is a response to the crises by dealing with uncertainty. Normally society would exert a moral power over the individual through regulation of human needs and desires. However, crises, be they positive or negative, can cause the society to become incapable of exercising regulation over individuals. It is for this reason that suicides increase. If homicide and suicide are seen as two sides of the same coin, suicide attacks and suicide bombing reflect the chaos in the society related to social changes, as the values and needs of both the society and the individual, especially those who are alienated, may change abruptly. This can take time to change the shape and regulation through what Durkheim calls *anomie*. In the world of trade and industry, Durkheim argues that there is a constant state of crisis and anomie. In capitalism in general and neo-liberal capitalism in particular, there is a constant state of crisis and anomie. On the one hand, religion has lost most of its power; on the other hand, nations have become preoccupied with industrial growth and GDP (gross domestic product). Although capitalism is sold as a success by the politicians, even communism is not free from this. Anomie is a regular and specific factor in causing suicide in our modern societies. Anomic suicide is different from the previous two types in that "it does not depend on the way in which individuals are attached to society, but on the way in which they are regulated by society." Therefore, minority youth may feel controlled and may respond in a more explosive manner. Furthermore, anomie can be seen in a number of situations and settings. Divorce in marital settings can be seen as an expression of this type of anomie, which consists of a weakening of "matrimonial regulation."

Religious Discovery

The word fanatic derives from Latin *fanum*, meaning someone who suffered from temple madness. Similarly, the term zealot is said to derive from a Jewish sect who fought against the Romans in the first century. Phillips and Ano reported from a sample of college students that religious fundamentalism was associated with a number of religious coping strategies, especially in cases of poor self-esteem and isolation and feelings of powerlessness.[19] It is possible that religious fundamentalism is a defense mechanism. Others have identified four coping strategies[20,21]: first, religious fundamentalism provides a sense of meaning and coherence to life. Second, fundamentalists are isolationists with clear rules to follow (which also provide a structure), thus coping better by using differences to mark religious boundaries. Third, extreme orthodoxy is seen as cleaning sins (also called purification), especially when faced with stress. And fourth, it is coping at an individual level without involving God. At times of uncertainty (equivalent to the anomie described by Durkheim), identity confusion and fear of perceived and real assaults on the vulnerable youth may lead to exploring fundamental ideologies perhaps to validate their own identity. Such a phenomenon is normative in adolescence when political idealism motivates youth to seek a place in the world, but usually this does not progress to acts of crime.

Durkheim deals with the origins of religions in his book *The Elementary Forms of the Religious Life*,[22] and argues that religion is social and has a collective representation that acts as cohesion of the in-group. It could be seen as social capital. Religious rites and rituals are seen as matters of acting which occur within the assembled groups. Religious beliefs can be both simple and complex, but the underlying theme is the possibly strong distinction between the sacred and the profane. In this context, sacred is what the interdictions protect and isolate, whereas profanities are the things to which interdictions are applied. Religious beliefs should be seen as representations which express the nature of sacred things and the relations which they have with each other or with profane things. Rites and rituals dictate how human beings should behave in the presence of sacred objects. With a decline in religious practice in many countries it is entirely possible that the younger generation are looking for an understanding and meaning and purpose of life and belonging. McTernan suggests that religious extremists often see themselves as "interpreters of history," believing that they alone have the knowledge to direct the course of events.[23] They see themselves as "the chosen ones" with an inalienable right to interpret divine revelation in a given circumstance. Selective in their tradition, heritage, and use of sacred texts, they have a worldview characterized by an uncompromising dualism of good versus bad and reject relativism and individualism as threats to identity.

It is important to recognize that normlessness may well underlie a lack of sense of purpose, as Dean recognizes that these are feelings of purposelessness and conflict of norms[24] (defined by De Grazia as being between cooperation and competition or between the "activist" and the "quietist" actions[25]). Social isolation may further contribute to the sense of normlessness, but it can be difficult to ascertain which comes first: whether social isolation leads to alienation, or is a result of some basic personality traits that encourage isolation and withdrawal which can then lead to alienation, is difficult to judge. The social isolation hypothesis (Jaco, 1954 cited in Dean[24]) argues that in residential areas with higher rates of schizophrenia there are high levels of anonymity, lower percentage of voting, greater unemployment and low social participation, higher rates of job turnover, and fewer visits with friends. Dean argues that there is a negative correlation between social status and alienation (in this context, social status was defined as level of education and income).[24] He concludes that alienation may be a situation-relevant variable rather than a personality trait, which provides an opportunity to develop public mental health interventions.

Vega et al. studied acculturation levels and delinquent behaviors among Cuban American adolescents and produced an empirical model.[26] These authors also studied protective family factors and a disposition to deviance while linking cultural conflict and acculturation. They proposed that deviance, like acculturation, is another concept with roots in the study of immigrants and their cultural and social adjustments. Arguably, deviance can be socially determined as well as socially transmitted. There are possibilities for genetic or biological factors. Social learning theory has been used to explain deviance.[27] Social structures appear to have a direct effect on psychological well-being and social behavior.[28] Merton postulated that the impact of unequal access to opportunity and achievement in the structures of society can then lead to a "structured strain" among (vulnerable) individuals who may seek rewards from society through non-normative means.[28] There is no doubt that differential acculturation across generations of migrants to the new society may undermine parental authority and family communication. Adolescents and young men in particular may face culture conflict on two fronts—with their parents and with the larger new culture. The individual's response by becoming deviant should therefore be understood in that context. The rejection of the new norms from the new culture and the old norms from parents and family places the vulnerable individual at a high risk for developing alienations and thereafter becoming deviant. Therefore, adolescents who are caught up in the personal and social dynamic of acculturation are at unusual risk for a variety of personal and social adjustment problems including non-normative deviant behavior.[26] Minority and immigrant status may well contribute to poor functioning and alienation, especially among vulnerable individuals. Strong family ties and personal attachments may therefore go on to mitigate these problems. Vega et al. go on to postulate that a tendency to social deviance can be potentiated if family protective factors are absent.[26] People typically behave in order to minimize the experience of self-rejecting attitudes and maximize the experience of positive self-attitudes.[29]

This model of rejection and derogation means that adolescents change their behavior in order to satisfy their parents' expectation, so their disapproval may lead to personal distress. The same also applies to teachers. However, Vega et al. pointed out that if either adolescents do not change their behavior or are simply unable to change negative assessments, this may lead to a disposition to deviance.[26] Such a disposition in the Kaplan et al.

model can lead to deviant peer group affiliation and ultimately to delinquent behaviors.[29]

Using this as their basis, Vega et al. explored whether acculturation and family protection factors might play a role in a disposition to deviance and delinquency.[26] Their data confirmed that family variables are important for creating vulnerability and, once that has been created, then acculturation strain variables have a stronger role in producing the actual behavior. Family conflict itself may be part of the acculturation process and may lead to individual vulnerability. Vega et al. recommend that intergenerational conflicts between adolescents and parents, financial pressures, parental disputes, spousal or child abuse, and substance abuse in the family contribute to a disposition and vulnerability to deviance.[26] For women it raises different questions. Fatani has argued that "the romantic element in the pitch for women in the Western countries is bolstered by a discourse of empowerment by showing that the recruit will be valued and important in an organization that portrays itself in stereotypically masculine characteristics as strong and protective".[30]

Social Integration and Radicalization

Berkman et al.,[31] by using Durkheim's social integration and attachment theories, argue that the social networks influence social support, social engagement, social influence, and access to resources. Barnes[32] and Bott[33] developed the notion of social network to describe traditional kinships, residential and other groups to describe behaviors which may feed into individual's functioning, such as jobs, political activities, etc. Analyzing networks allows us to focus on characteristic patterns of relationships and ties between individuals within that specific network and how this impinges upon their functioning. Hall and Wellman pointed out that social network analysis looks at not only structures and composition of networks, but also its strengths.[34] Both egocentric and complete networks require exploration to understand an individual member's social functioning. The core of the community is formed of these social networks and structures that may well influence the in-groups as well as the out-groups.

The link between alienation and not belonging on the one hand and belonging on the other with low levels of culture conflict need further detailed exploration. Our conjecture is that a sense of alienation may be triggered by any number of factors and may therefore be compounded by culture conflict and contribute to deviance and delinquency presenting as violent radicalization which provides individuals a sense of being and belonging. Furthermore, the absence of strong family ties or conflict with majority culture may push the vulnerable individual towards embracing deviant acts which give them a sense of purpose as well as of belonging. Our model is illustrated in Figure 3.1.

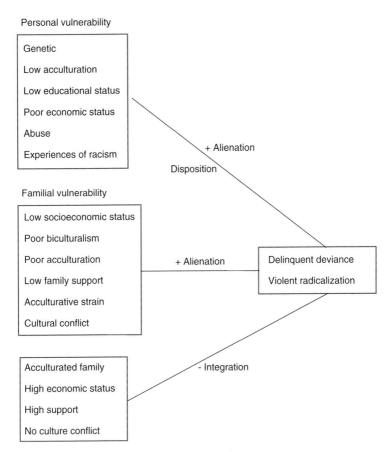

Figure 3.1. Protective and contributive causative factors.

As discussed elsewhere,[35] it is possible that violent attacks may be seen as a result of mental illness rather than pure terrorist activity. Psychiatrists and mental health professionals have been asked for centuries to assess risk and manage risk related to the mental state of perpetrators and also to play a role in understanding the causes of violent radicalization.

Violent radicalization is put forward as a result of religious fundamentalism, and this contested position has led to stigmatization of migrants and especially people of Muslim heritage born and brought up in Western democracies. This focus has often been part of political and governmental debates that insist on possible solutions against radicalization based on nationalist values and nationalist identity and that migrants must swear allegiance to the leaders of Western democracies. This culturally constructed and optimistic intervention resonates with the voice of the political right, a movement that is becoming increasingly louder and prominent not only in Europe but also in the USA and some parts of Asia. The expectation is that individuals give up their cultural views and become homogenized after migration, or be returned to their countries of origin irrespective of the situations they may have escaped from. Similar arguments are rehearsed at times of natural disaster or war and conflict when asylum is sought by people fleeing these hazards.

Prevention of Terror

The cultural war on terrorism not only attacks the narratives of radical movements, but their arguments play into the hands of so-called terrorists. The policy-makers in turn go on to assert that preventive paradigms and interventions, if applied early, can lead to the prevention of terrorist actions. For example, in the UK, classroom teaching on extremism for school children is now mandatory. The responsibility falls not only on teachers, but also on psychiatrists and mental health professionals to deliver prevention programs. There are obviously ethical and professional dilemmas for a number of reasons. For example, risk assessment is valid only for short periods and as mental health professionals cannot predict risk, it is difficult to predict potential for terrorist activities. This science of prediction for rare events is poor in adults and even weaker in adolescents and school children.

Psychotic depression has been implicated rather than mild depression in acts of aggression.[36–39] Social isolation has also been shown to play a role in providing a plausible link between psychological, social, and criminal experiences in radicalization.[40]

As Lamy et al. remind us,[41] that small groups may face existential uncertainty easily, even if larger studies are needed on how psychological factors, within groups, may facilitate group acculturation. The concepts related to ethno-cultural continuity, defined as the process by which ethno-cultural groups as heterogeneous living entities retain their uniqueness while undergoing change as they travel through time (socio-historical contexts) and space (larger societies), are important in the context of both the in-group and the out-group. Weinreich (p. 128) considers this sense of ethnicity as variously held in the imagination and sustained by societal artifacts of the ethnic culture in question, but also the reality and this tension between held ethnicity and perception can be seen as a critical step in understanding religious fundamentalism.[42] Cultural continuity reflects both the past and the history and the future, but maintains symbolic and cultural heritage.[43]

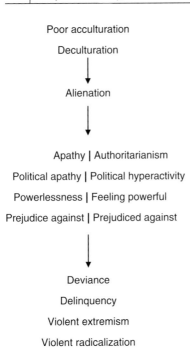

Poor acculturation

Deculturation

Alienation

Apathy | Authoritarianism

Political apathy | Political hyperactivity

Powerlessness | Feeling powerful

Prejudice against | Prejudiced against

Deviance

Delinquency

Violent extremism

Violent radicalization

Figure 3.2. Relationship between alienation as a result of poor acculturation or due to culture conflict.

Therefore, an exploration of the cultural identity of the third generation at the identity level, both at a group level and at an individual level, becomes critical. Anecdotally, it appears that the first generation tries to assimilate and straddle two cultures, whereas in the second generation the likelihood of culture conflict becomes more important. The third generation may feel further isolated and look for identity, especially in the context of continuity of what their parents and grandparents may have gone through. We believe that the way of exploring alienation is to study social factors that will have a major implication to create public mental health interventions (Figure 3.2 illustrates the relationship between alienation as a result of poor acculturation or due to culture conflict).

A smaller proportion of people who may be self-selected or vulnerable may be at risk, so that an even smaller portion will carry out violent acts. The factors for violent radicalization at a macro-level will include political aspects, geo-political factors, public opinion, and government actions and political parties who may fuel violent radicalization. At micro-level racism, discrimination, challenges to identity, social isolation, poverty, lack of or poor acculturation and mental ill health may contribute.

Essential steps and strategies in managing violent radicalization are: safety, calming, coping possibilities, enhancing group cohesion, and instilling hope.

Conclusions

Any sense of alienation and of not belonging in the face of culture conflict may well play a significant role in developing deviant behavior and consequent participation in gang culture to develop one's identity, which may then progress to violent radicalization. A mixture of cultural and public health approaches are indicated not only to understand these pathways, but also to put preventive measures in place. Religion and religious fanaticism combined with political hyperactivity as a result of alienation may prove to be a potent mixture leading to a sense of belonging by joining gangs and indulging in potentially damaging and destructive behavior. Poor political engagement, along with a sense of alienation, religious conversion or new religious interests, and adverse acculturative outcome predispose individuals to social isolation and vulnerability to a number of adverse health outcomes. These outcomes may include radicalization and terrorism; but what drives people down this path rather than gang membership, drug use, or other types of offending is yet to be discerned and deserves urgent attention.

References

1. Marks, S, Pick, D. Lessons on mind control from the 1950s. *The World Today*. 2017; Feb/March: 14–16.

2. Redfield, R, Linton, R, Herskovitz, MJ. Memorandum for the study of acculturation. *Am Anthropol*. 1936; **38**: 149–152.

3. Berry, J. Acculturation and identity. In: Bhugra D, Bhui K, eds. *Textbook of Cultural Psychiatry*. Cambridge: Cambridge University Press; 2018: 185–193.

4. Graves, TD. Acculturation, access, and alcohol in a tri-ethnic community. *Am Anthropol*. 1967; **69**(3–4): 306–321.

5. Berry, J. Acculturation as varieties of adaptation. In: Padilla A, ed. *Acculturation: Theory, Models and Findings*. Boulder, CO: Westview; 1980: 9–25.

6. Berry, J. Acculturation and adaptation in a new society. *Int Migration*. 1992; **30**: 69–85.

7. Berry, J. Immigration, acculturation and adaptation. *Appl Psychol*. 1997; **46**: 5–68.

8. Berry, J, Kim, U. Comparative stresses of acculturative stress. *Int Migration Rev*. 1987; **21**: 491–511.

9. Hajda, J. Alienation and integration of student intellectuals. *Am Sociol Rev*. 1961; **26** (5): 758–777.

10. Keniston, K. Alienation and decline of Utopia. *Am Scholar*. 1960; **29**: 164.

11. Adorno, TW, Brunswick-Frenkel, E, Levinson, D, Sanford, N. *The Authoritarian Personality*. New York, NY: Harper & Brothers; 1950: 618.

12. Rosenberg, M. The meaning of politics in mass society. *Publ Opin Quart*. 1951; **15**: 5–15.

13. Riesman, D, Glazer, N. Criteria for political apathy. In: Gouldner AW, ed. *Studies in Leadership*. New York, NY: Harper & Brothers; 1950: 505–559.

14. Marcuse, H. *Reason and Revolution*. New York, NY: Oxford University Press; 1941: 34.

15. Powell, E. Occupation, status and suicide: towards a redefinition of anomie. *Am Sociol Rev*. 1953; **23**: 131–139.

16. Manne, A. Narcissism and terrorism: how the personality disorder leads to deadly violence. *The Guardian*, 8 June 2015.

17. Durkheim, E. *On Suicide*, trans. J. Spaulding, G. Simpson. Glencoe, IL: Free Press; 1897/1951: 246–258.

18. Olsen, ME. Durkheim's two concepts of anomie. *Sociol Quart*. 1965; **6**: 37–44.

19. Phillips, RE, Ano, GG. A re-examination of religious fundamentalism: positive implications for coping. *Mental Hlth Relig Culture*. 2015; **18**: 299–311.

20. Herriot, P. *Religious Fundamentalism and Social Identity*. New York, NY: Routledge; 2007.

21. Hood, RW, Hill, PC, Williamson, WP. *The Psychology of Religious Fundamentalism*. New York, NY: Guilford Press; 2005.

22. Durkheim, E. *The Elementary Forms of the Religious Life*, trans. C. Cosman. Oxford: Oxford University Press; 1915/2006.

23. McTernen, O. Let us not prey. *The World Today*. 2017; Feb/Mar: 21–22.

24. Dean, DG. Alienation: its meaning and measurement. *Am Sociol Rev*. 1961; **26**(5): 753–758.

25. De Grazia, S. *The Political Community: A Study of Anomies*. Chicago, IL: University of Chicago Press; 1948: 8–20, 115–122.

26. Vega, WA, Gil, AG, Warheit, GJ, Zimmerman, RS, Apospori, E. Acculturation and delinquent behaviour among Cuban American adolescents: toward an empirical model. *Am J Community Psychol*. 1993; **21**: 113–125.

27. Sutherland, EH. *Principles of Criminology*. Philadelphia, PA: Lippincott; 1939.

28. Merton, RK. Social structure and anomie. *Am Sociol Rev*. 1938; **3**: 672–682.

29. Kaplan, H, Johnson, R, Bailey, C. Self rejection and the explanation of deviance: refinement and elaboration of a latent structure. *Social Psychol Quart*. 1986; **49**: 110–128.

30. Fatani, S. Wooing the jihadi brides. *The World Today*. 2017; Feb/Mar: 23.

31. Berkman, L, Glass, T, Brissette, I, Seeman, T. From social integration to health: Durkheim in the new millennium. *Soc Sci & Med*. 2000; **51**: 843–857.

32. Barnes, JA. Class and committees in a Norwegian island parish. *Human Relations*. 1954; **7**: 39–58.

33. Bott, E. *Family and Social Network*. London: Tavistock; 1957.

34. Hall, A, Wellman, B. Social networks and social support. In: Cohen S, Syme SL, eds. *Social Support and Health*. Orlando, FL: Academic Press; 1985: 23–41.

35. Bhugra, D, Ventriglio, A, Bhui, KS. Acculturation, violent radicalisation and religious fundamentalism. *Lancet Psychiatry*. 2017; **4**: 179–181.

36. Victoroff, J. The mind of the terrorist: a review and critique of psychological approaches. *J Conflict Resol*. 2005; **49**: 3–42.

37. Victoroff, J, Quota, S, Adelman, JR, Celinska, B, Stern, N, et al. Support for religio-political aggression among teenage boys in Gaza. Part 1: Psychological findings. *Aggress Behav*. 2010; **36**: 219–231.

38. Bénézech, M, Bourgeois, M. Homicide is strongly correlated to depression and not to mania. *Encephale*. 1992; **18**(Spec No. 1): 89–90.

39. Osipova, DV, Kulikov, A, Popova, NK. C1473 G polymorphism in mouse *tph2* gene is limited to tryptophan hydroxylase-2 activity in the brain, inter male aggression and depressive-like behaviour in the forced swim test. *J Neurosci Res*. 2009; **87**: 1168–1174.

40. McCauley, C, Moskalenko, M. *Friction: How Radicalization Happens to Them and Us*. New York, NY: Oxford University Press; 2011: 248.

41. Lamy, MAG, Ward, C, Liu, JH. Motivation for ethno-cultural continuity. *J Cross-Cult Psychol*. 2013; **44**: 1047.

42. Weinreich, P. "Enculturation" not "acculturation": conceptualising and assessing identity processes in migrant communities. *Int J Intercult Rel*. 2009; **33**: 124–139.

43. Verkuyten, M. *The Social Psychology of Ethnic Identity*. Hove: Psychology Press; 2005.

Chapter

4

The Mind of Suicide Terrorists

Donatella Marazziti, Antonello Veltri, and
Armando Piccinni

Introduction

The number of terrorist attacks, particularly those carried out by suicide
bombers, also called modern kamikazes, is dramatically increasing worldwide.
Since 1995, the year of the attack on the American Embassy in Beirut,
considered by many to be the first of this type of terrorist act, more than
70,000 attacks have been completed, which have killed 170,000 and wounded
300,000. Modern suicide terrorism has some peculiarities.[1,2] First, this phenomenon is no longer confined to the countries of the Middle East, traditionally characterized by political instability, but now occurs throughout the
world. Second, the most recent attacks in Western countries have been
perpetrated by first- or second-generation immigrants raised according to
local rules and educated in local schools, who suddenly, at some point in
their personal trajectory, embraced religious radicalization and repudiated the
values of their societies. It is now evident that every country, every activity, and
every person not sharing their beliefs and values are potential targets. Third, if
previous terrorist activities were characterized and motivated by more or less
declared political aims (e.g., the Red Brigades in Italy, the Rote Armee
Fraktion in Germany, and the IRA in Ireland),[3–8] the latest suicidal attacks
are driven by religion and carried out by extremists who claim to serve as
God's instruments to destroy the West, which they consider impure and
corrupted.[9,10] This is crucial, because it implies that these terrorists are
(perhaps) not afraid to die, or at least they do not show any reluctance about
abandoning their lives while at the same time killing innocent victims, without
any apparent regret or overt emotionality. Instead of the joy of life or plans for
a creative and better future, they harbor and fuel hatred for the members of
their society, and they cultivate the concept of martyrdom and worship death,
expecting to be rewarded in paradise.[11] To further complicate the situation,
the attacks in Western countries over the last couple of years appear totally
different from those of the past, with the apparent waning of a "central"
strategy and even strict religious motivations, as they are now mainly perpetrated by isolated individuals, the so-called "lone wolves," claiming to have
acted on behalf of the so-called Islamic State (ISIL).

There are three essential questions that all professionals (including psychologists, psychiatrists, and neuroscientists) involved in understanding and possibly preventing terrorism should try to answer:

1. Who are the modern suicide terrorists?
2. What are they: psychopaths, psychiatric patients, personality-disordered subjects, or something else?
3. Why does someone become a terrorist, and what are the psychological processes that drive an individual to become a lethal weapon?

The answer to the third question is the key to disentangling a crucial quandary: how is it possible that an individual would choose to deliberately die in order to kill someone else?

In the 1970s, these questions were mainly approached using sociological and political explanations.[12–14] During the next two decades, much attention was paid to psychological or psychosocial factors,[15–20] with the result pointed out by Victoroff[21] that "the number of suggested theories far outstrips the number of empirical studies in the literature." These hypotheses were soon generally discredited. Instead of the previous rigid categorizations, there was a series of novel and creative suggestions that, though suicide terrorists do not suffer from any specific personality disorders, they are nevertheless "peculiar." However, it should be underlined that the research in this area is complicated by difficulties in carrying out reliable studies with standardized instruments to "measure" and assess the suicidal terrorism phenomenon and the characteristics of terrorists. As a result, the available data appear to be not only heterogeneous and controversial, but also of limited value, since they were gathered in such small samples. According to John Horgan,[22] even more dangerous is the fact that the research on recent terrorism seems to neglect previous data and the caveats they present.

Further, we cannot ignore that the research in this field may be slowed down by the reluctance that some ferocious behaviors provoke in professionals, even mental health and brain specialists or criminologists, when faced with such cold evil that has no apparent purpose other than to frighten people. In any case, if some phenomena are present, recurrent, and of great impact, if they threaten our lives, our future, our world, and our way of living, they need to be approached correctly and understood as fully as possible, though they may evoke disgust, condemnation, and disapproval.[23]

The aim of our paper is to review the available literature in order to put forward some considerations and possible hypotheses on what could be the common psychological denominators or features shared by suicide terrorists and on what constitutes the "terrorist's mind."

Who and What Are the Terrorists?

Demographic studies from the 1960s and 1970s depicted a typical terrorist as a well-educated single male in his 20s and with a middle- or upper-class background.[12] Examining Federal Bureau of Investigation data on active terrorists in the United States during the 1960s and 1970s, it was found that female sex and completion of college were more common among left- than right-wing terrorists, while a blue-collar occupation was more common among right-wing terrorists.[13] Similar findings were obtained from investigations of Italian terrorists, where the women were reported to be predominantly in their 20s and mainly teachers or white-collar workers.[24] No significant differences in terms of family background were detected in a controlled study[25] comparing Italian Red Brigade members to politically active control subjects.

A change in the terrorist's profile was observed in the 1980s, when American and European revolutionary anarchist groups were becoming more quiescent and radical Islamic terrorism was growing worldwide. The typical Palestinian terrorists of this period were initially and uniformly described as aged 17 to 23 years, coming from large and impoverished families, and having low levels of education.[26] Subsequent studies, however, yielded different data. Sageman[27] reported that more than 70 per cent of Muslim terrorists had a college education and that more than 50 per cent were professionals. As he wrote in 2004, "These are the best and brightest of their societies in many ways." Krueger and Maleckova[27] compared a group of Hezbollah fighters with members of the general Lebanese population of the same age range and showed that the poverty rate was similar, but that the fighters were significantly more likely to have attended secondary school. Such reports were clearly inconsistent with the theories matching radical Islamic terrorists with poverty and a lack of education.[28] Currently, it is clear that Middle Eastern terrorists from the late 1990s came from a wider demographic range, including university students, professionals, married men in their late 40s, and even young women.[29] From a recent revision of one of his previous studies,[4] Merari,[30] analyzing and comparing 15 suicide bombers and 14 recruiters with 12 non-suicide terrorists, concluded that the former had higher educational and economic levels, higher religiosity, and were suffering more frequently from avoidant and dependent personality disorders, and sometimes from depression.[4,30]

Other personality traits commonly reported and proposed in the literature include narcissism, paranoia, victimization, and psychopathy.[31-34] In any case, if the motivations of a typical psychopath are complex and involve personalized fantasies, both suicide bombers and psychopaths would seem to lack social and moral constraints, and they explicitly refuse the conventional moral limits that are generally accepted during times of war.[35] In any case, the data supporting psychopathy or sociopathy as important features of the psychology of terrorism are limited, but there is no reason that terrorist groups should be considered organizations of psychopathic individuals because of the brutality of their behavior, nor do they predominantly recruit psychopaths.[36] On the contrary, some data indicate that terrorist leaders generally refuse to accept unstable individuals, who may become a danger to the group. Interestingly, even Hassan-i-Sabbah, the founder and grandmaster of the *Hashshashin* (Assassins), avoided recruiting for murderers those adepts who became agitated after smoking hashish. However, there is no doubt that suicide bombers show cold cruelty, no empathy, nor any sense of pity or guilt about their deeds, similar to sociopathic individuals. But they are not necessarily sociopaths.[23]

Why Does Somebody Become a Terrorist?

If suicide terrorists do not meet the diagnostic criteria for personality disorders, major psychiatric disorders, or for psychopathy, what can explain their violent and immoral behavior? According to the so-called "rational choice theory," terrorist actions derive from a calculated decision or strategy intended to accomplish sociopolitical goals:[37,38] to perpetrate violence and engender fear.

However, there is evidence which suggests that *very* few subjects, even those who support the goals of terrorists, ever become suicide terrorists.[39] This theory thus fails to explain why only a small minority of such individuals end up as terrorists. If neither psychopathology/psychopathy nor rationality account for the genesis of terrorist behavior, what alternative explanations exist? In the past few decades, a lot of sociological and psychological theories have been proposed, but none can be considered valid and reliable. As reviewed by Victoroff,[21] these theories are categorized as sociological theories, psychoanalytic psychological theories, nonpsychoanalytic psychological theories, and group process theories (Table 4.1).

Some very interesting speculations may derive from a 1997 Canadian study, in which 1,482 university students (629 men and 853 women) were analyzed to deepen our understanding of the characteristics of individuals who answered "yes" to the statement "If God told me to kill, I would do it in His name."[40] The odds ratio of an affirmative response for men and women was 1.4/1. Other factors significantly associated with an affirmative response included weekly church attendance, a history of a religious experience, and elevated complex partial epileptic-like signs (limbic lability). If generalizable, these findings, as proposed by the author, would suggest that "one out of every 20 university men would be willing to kill another person" if God instructed him to do so. It is conceivable that such elements may represent risk factors for the engagement of young students with terrorist groups. It can

Table 4.1 Sociological and psychological theories of terrorism

Sociological theories		
Social learning theory of aggression	Teaching or social learning may influence some young people toward terrorism	Bandura (1998a,b)[a]
Frustration–aggression hypothesis	The terrorist violent acts are interpreted as a reaction to desperation, frustration, and oppression	Dollard et al. (1939)[b] Davies (2003)[c]
Relative deprivation theory	Either absolute deprivation or relative economic disparity provoke terrorist sentiments among members of an oppressed underclass	Gurr (1970)[d]
Psychoanalytic psychological theories		
Identity theory	Candidates for terrorism are young people lacking self-esteem who have strong needs to consolidate their identities	Olsson (1988)[e] Ferracuti (1982)[f]
Narcissism theory	Political experience such as humiliation or subordination may produce an adult narcissistic injury which brings to light an infantile one (damage to self-image due to poor maternal care)	Crayton (1983)[g] Shaw (1986)[h]
Paranoia theory	The terrorist has suspicions that justify bloody acts of "self-defense" against his victims	Robins and Post (1997)[i]
Absolutist/apocalyptic theory	In absolutist groups, moral polarization and idealization of a messianic figure may motivate terrorism in young adults with weak identities	Lifton (2000)[j]
Nonpsychoanalytic psychological theories		
Cognitive theories	Some cognitive errors (attribution errors) and a peculiar cognitive style (inflexibility) may represent a general trait of terrorists	Taylor (1988)[k] Sidanius (1985)[l]
Novelty-seeking theory	Terrorist violent acts may satisfy innate and genetically determined needs for high-level stimulation and risk	Kellen (1979)[m] Levine (1999)[n]

Table 4.1 (cont.)

Nonpsychoanalytic psychological theories		
Humiliation–revenge theory	Humiliation by an oppressor and the consequent internal pressure for revenge can be a psychological factor capable of driving terrorist violence	Juergensmeyer (2000)[o]

Theories of group process		
	Group forces—including ideological indoctrination, repetitive training, and peer pressures—may drive the group's violence, whether or not individual members are predisposed for such behavior	Crenshaw (1992)[p] Clayton et al. (1998)[q]

[a] Bandura, A. Health promotion from the perspective of social cognitive theory. *Psychol Health*. 1998a; **13**: 623–649. Bandura A. Mechanisms of moral disengagement. In: Reich W, ed. *Origins of Terrorism: Psychologies, Ideologies, Theologies, States of Mind*. Washington, DC: Woodrow Wilson Center Press; 1998b: 161–192.

[b] Dollard, J, Doob, LW, Miller, NE, Mowrer, OB, Sears, RR. *Frustration and Aggression*. New Haven, CT: Yale University Press; 1939.

[c] Davies, B. *Terrorism: Inside a World Phenomenon*. London: Virgin Books; 2003.

[d] Gurr, TR. *Why Men Rebel*. Princeton, NJ: Princeton University Press; 1970.

[e] Olsson, PA. The terrorist and the terrorized: some psychoanalytic consideration. *J Psychohist*. 1988; **16** (1): 47–60.

[f] Ferracuti, F. A sociopsychiatric interpretation of terrorism. *Ann Am Acad Polit Soc Sci*. 1982; **463**: 129–140.

[g] Crayton, JW. Terrorism and the psychology of the self. In: Freedman AZ, Alexander Y, eds. *Perspectives on Terrorism*. Wilmington, DE: Scholarly Resources; 1983: 33–41.

[h] Shaw, ED. Political terrorists: dangers of diagnosis and an alternative to the psychopathological model. *Int J Law Psychiatry*. 1986; **8**(3): 359–366.

[i] Robins, RS, Post, JM. *Political Paranoia: The Psychopolitics of Hatred*. New Haven, CT: Yale University Press; 1997.

[j] Lifton, RJ. 2000. *Destroying the World to Save It: Aum Shinrikyo and the New Global Terrorism*. New York: Holt; 2000.

[k] Taylor, M. *The Terrorist*. London: Brassey's; 1988.

[l] Sidanius, J. Cognitive functioning and sociopolitical ideology revisited. *Polit Psychol*. 1985; **6**: 637–666.

[m] Kellen, K. *Terrorists—What Are They Like? How Some Terrorists Describe Their World and Actions*. Santa Monica, CA: Rand; 1979.

[n] Levine, S. Youths in terroristic groups, gangs and cults: the allure, the animus, and the alienation. *Psychiatr Ann*. 1999; **29**: 342–349.

[o] Juergensmeyer, M. *Terror in the Mind of God*. Berkeley: University of California Press; 2000.

[p] Crenshaw, M. How terrorists think: what psychology can contribute to understanding terrorism. In: Howard L, ed. *Terrorism: Roots, Impact, Responses*. New York: Praeger; 1992: 71–80.

[q] Clayton, SV. Preference for macrojustice vs. microjustice in environmental decisions. *Environ Behav*. 1998; **30**: 162–183.

be hypothesized that a less flexible cognitive style in men with respect to women could confer susceptibility to maintain orthodoxy and exclude (negate) some elements of reflection, such as the long-term consequences of their actions. Again, it is conceivable that extreme behaviors may be acted out within peculiar social, political, and historical contexts, as shown in a previous study in the United States,[41] or in times of social uncertainty.[42] When paralleled and sustained by religious beliefs elicited by charismatic leaders, as in the case of modern kamikazes, this mix is deadly. The role of charismatic leaders is important in this sense, as they fuel the original sense of humiliation, typical of individuals who harbor a sense of not belonging to their society. Such leaders employ their authority to elicit homicidal impulses. Research on the personality of such leaders highlighted their extroversion, egocentrism, and lack of emotionality, but also critical refusal, suspiciousness, and aggression.[43] Adherence to religious rituals and shared intents is almost always associated with social rewards from a community, and this could strengthen a sense of belonging and an individual's identification with the aims and beliefs of a terrorist group. Some studies have focused on the power of religion as a tool to bring fulfillment to an empty life, especially when the values transmitted by an individual's original families are lost or have been repudiated by the individual, in order to fuel acceptance by his/her compatriots. This process frequently fosters an increasing sense of isolation that can be compensated for and resolved by religion and/or belonging to a group where the individuals feel that they have become an important tile in the mosaic, that they have been appointed for a precise mission. Religious experiences are heterogeneous events in which a person feels an emotional peak, feels the presence of God, or has lucid dreams and ecstatic moments of inspiration.[44] These sensations are associated with other signs of limbic lability, including subthreshold temporal epileptic phenomena, particularly of the right brain. Since the limbic system plays such a crucial role in the integration of emotions and thoughts, functional abnormalities therein may allow for a particular emotional state that interferes with higher cognitive processes. Finally, religious experiences and other events associated with limbic lability can influence an individual's choices while introducing new priorities in their life.[44,45] In this way, terrorism provides isolated individuals with a motivation where the related actions and their bloody consequences *are* the reward.

Conclusions

The impact of suicide terrorist attacks is enormous and has produced significant changes in the everyday life of Western nations. Though such acts are much less common than in such regions as the Middle East, the West has become a more common target. Unfortunately, though it may be comforting to infer that suicide bombers may suffer from personality/psychiatric disorders, or are psychopaths, the available data, including those gathered by an expert committee organized some years ago, suggest that modern kamikazes are not mentally ill.[19,22,23,46,47] However, it is evident that their cruel behavior and the motivations behind them have nothing to do with what any individual with a conscience would consider normal. For these reasons, aside from political, sociological, and economical considerations, it is essential that some attempts should be made to bring together some of the widely recognized characteristics of suicide bombers in order to outline how it is possible that apparently normal individuals can behave in these unacceptable ways, as well as to trace possible hypotheses about which of their psychological processes would suggest a sort of particular "mind of a suicide terrorist." Obviously, without neglecting the contributions of past studies,[22] in spite of all their limitations, and while highlighting how it might be reductionist to try and put together different features of a phenomenon that is so multifaceted and increasingly heterogeneous, it could be important to study small samples of regretful, failed, or intercepted terrorists.

Let us start from what we consider the core of terrorist behavior. According to us, this is constituted by the reversal of one of the most important, if not the main, human instinct—to survive, to live. In suicide bombers, this instinct seems to be totally replaced by the death instinct, with the specific connotation that it is rewarding to die while killing many others. "To die to kill" is certainly ethically unacceptable, unintelligible if not included within a type of thinking that is "abnormal" without being pathological, as the literature suggests,[19,20,22,23,30,46–48] which perhaps should be more correctly defined as "extranormal," or at least very far away from that domain that we consider "normality." When there is an inversion of the common value of "life over death" in favor of "death over life," some other psychological changes may soon occur. Life is no longer appealing, not only one's own, but also that of thousands of innocent bystanders. Aside from that, the suicide terrorist develops (probably instigated by the group leader and by a type of negative group therapy focusing on extreme religious values and revenge for past wrongs)[36] a sort of lust for or addiction to martyrdom and death,[9–11] even promoted by a basic (or drug-induced in some cases) disturbance of the reward system and altered dopamine neurotransmission.[49] Who cares if one's current life is bad? The martyr will go to paradise after death and after murdering those who do not share the same religious values.

Along these lines, it should not be too surprising that suicide terrorists seem to lack some important features of humanity and characteristics of human sociability when acting out in ferocious ways that shock us, with a feral bravery amplified by sophisticated usage of new technologies. That is why their aim is not only to kill people (even children and adolescents returning home after a concert in Manchester or traveling in a bus to attend a religious service in Egypt, just to name a few of the latest attacks), but to destroy the symbols of Western decadence (e.g., discotheques, arenas, and restaurants), and the edifices and symbols of the Christian faith. However, more importantly, they wish to elicit worldwide dread and insecurity. At the basis of this behavior, there are both an indifference for others' suffering and a cultivated hatred for their peers and society in general.

All suicide terrorist actions, even those accomplished by lone wolves and carried out with less elaborate plans and weaponry, share the same cold rationality. This implies that terrorists are generally rational individuals able to consider the pros and cons of their behavior and its impact within a specific context. However, the considerations that lie at the basis of this behavioral rationality are clearly illogical, as they are derived via a profound alteration of cognitive processes and distortion of reality that could be considered "psychotic."[50] The excessive rationality coupled with extreme coldness resembles those clinical features described by Antonio Damasio[51] in several of his neurological patients who showed impairment of those parts of the brain involved in emotional processing (e.g., the limbic structures and their connections to other brain regions and the prefrontal cortex).[51] Without emotions, "man is not reasonable." It is only through a measured balance between emotions and reason that our humanity may spring forth.[52,53]

In terms of preventing suicide terrorism, aside from political and economic changes, from the psychological point of view, strong efforts need to be devoted to promoting and nourishing correct development of emotions in children and adolescents, especially those exposed to early traumas or who live in troubling situations. It is also mandatory to act at the level of the recruiters so as to reduce the psychological power they wield on their followers, so that these disciples can be rescued and returned to a "normal" life, where they could learn to appreciate shared human values and where they could learn to respect the laws that carry no religious connotations. Put in other words, as Sophocles had Antigone declare in his eponymous tragedy, these values and laws are embedded in our nature: "For their life is not of to-day or yesterday, but for all time, and no man knows when they were first put forth."[54]

Disclosures

Donatella Marazziti, Antonello Veltri, and Armando Piccinni hereby declare that they have conflicts of interest to disclose.

References

1. Lankford, A. Public opinions of suicide bombers' mental health. *Compr Psychol.* 2014; **3**: 15. http://journals.sagepub.com/doi/full/10.2466/07.CP.3.15. Accessed August 16, 2017.

2. Townsend, E. Suicide terrorists: are they suicidal? *Suicide Life Threat Behav.* 2007; **37** (1): 35–49.

3. Crenshaw, M. The causes of terrorism. *Comp Polit.* 1981; **13**: 379–399.

4. Merari, A. The readiness to kill and die: suicidal terrorism in the Middle East. In: Reich W, ed. *Origins of Terrorism: Psychologies, Ideologies, Theologies, States of Mind.* Washington, DC: Woodrow Wilson Center Press; 1998: 192–207.

5. Crenshaw, M. The psychology of political terrorism. In: Hermann MG, ed. *Political Psychology.* San Francisco: Jossey-Bass; 1986: 379–413.

6. Schmid, A. *Political Terrorism: A Research Guide to the Concepts, Theories, Databases and Literature,* with a bibliography by the author and a world directory of "terrorist" organizations by A.J. Jongman. Amsterdam: North Holland; 1983.

7. Blain, M. Social science discourse and the biopolitics of terrorism. *Sociol Compass.* 2015; **9**: 161–179.

8. Della Porta, D. Recruitment processes in clandestine political organizations: Italian left-wing terrorism. *Int Soc Mov Res.* 1988; **1**: 155–169.

9. Lankford, A. *The Myth of Martyrdom: What Really Drives Suicide Bombers, Rampage Shooters, and Other Self-Destructive Killers.* New York: St Martin's Press; 2014.

10. Gill, A. Religion and violence: an economic approach. In: Murphy AR, ed. *The Blackwell Companion to Religion and Violence.* Hoboken, NJ: Wiley-Blackwell; 2011: 35–49.

11. Sela, Y, Shackelford, TK. The myth of the myth of martyrdom. *Behav Brain Sci.* 2014; **37**(4): 376–377.

12. Russell, CA, Miller, BH. Profile of a terrorist. In: Freedman LZ, Alexander Y, eds. *Perspectives on Terrorism.* Wilmington, DE: Scholarly Resources; 1983: 45–60.

13. Handler, JS. Socioeconomic profile of an American terrorist: 1960s and 1970s. *Terrorism.* 1990; **13**: 195–213.

14. Atran, S. Genesis of suicide terrorism. *Science.* 2003; **299**(5612): 1534–1539.

15. Crenshaw, M. How terrorists think: what psychology can contribute to understanding terrorism. In: Howard L, ed. *Terrorism: Roots, Impact, Responses.* New York, NY: Praeger; 1992: 71–80.

16. Sageman, M. *Understanding Terror Networks.* Philadelphia, PA: University of Pennsylvania Press; 2004.

17. Post, JM, Sprinzak, E, Denny, LM. The terrorists in their own words: interviews with thirty-five incarcerated Middle Eastern terrorists. *Terror Polit Violence.* 2003; **15**: 171–184.

18. Ferracuti, F. A sociopsychiatric interpretation of terrorism. *Ann Am Acad Polit Soc Sci.* 1982; **463**: 129–140.

19. Post, JM, Ali, F, Henderson, SW, Shanfield, S, Victoroff, J, Weine, S. The psychology of suicide terrorism. *Psychiatry.* 2009; **72**(1): 13–31.

20. Post, JM. *The Mind of the Terrorist: The Psychology of Terrorism from the IRA to Al-Qaeda.* London: Palgrave Macmillan; 2007.

21. Victoroff, J. The mind of the terrorist. *J Conflict Resolut.* 2005; **49**(1): 3–42.

22. Horgan, J. *The Psychology of Terrorism.* Abingdon, UK: Routledge; 2014.

23. Marazziti, D. Psychiatry and terrorism: exploring the unacceptable. *CNS Spectr.* 2016; **21**(2): 128–130.

24. Weinberg, L, Eubank, WL. Italian women terrorists. *Terror Int J.* 1987; **9**: 241–262.

25. Ferracuti, F, Bruno, F. Psychiatric aspects of terrorism in Italy. In: Barak-Glantz IL, Huff CR, eds. *The Mad, the Bad and the Different: Essays in Honor of Simon Dinitz.* Lexington, MA: Lexington Books; 1981: 199–213.

26. Strentz, T. A terrorist psychosocial profile: past and present. *FBI Law Enforc Bull.* 1988; **57**: 13–19.

27. Krueger, AB, Maleckova, J. Education, poverty and terrorism: is there a causal connection? *J Econ Perspect.* 2003; **17**(4): 119–144.

28. Kaplan, A. The psychodynamics of terrorism. In: Alexander Y, Gleason J, eds. *Behavioral and Quantitative Perspectives on Terrorism.* New York, NY: Pergamon Press; 1981: 35–50.

29. Ripley, A. Why suicide bombing is now all the rage. *Time.* 2002; **159**(15): 33–39.

30. Merari, A. *Driven to Death: Psychological and Social Aspects of Suicide Terrorism.* New York, NY: Oxford Press; 2010.

31. Pearlstein, RM. *The Mind of a Political Terrorist.* Wilmington, DE: Scholarly Press; 1991.

32. Rasch, W. Psychological dimensions of political terrorism in the Federal Republic of Germany. *Int J Law Psychiatry.* 1979; **2**(1): 79–85.

33. Cooper, HHA. Psychopath as terrorist: a psychological perspective. *Leg Med Q.* 1978; **2**: 253–262.

34. Silke, AP. Cheshire-cat logic: the recurring theme of terrorist abnormality in psychological research. *Psychol Crime Law.* 1998; **4**: 51–69.

35. Blair, RJ. Applying a cognitive neuroscience perspective to the disorder of psychopathy. *Dev Psychopathol.* 2005; **17**(3): 865–891.

36. Post, JM. *Leaders and Their Followers in a Dangerous World: The Psychology of Political Behavior.* Ithaca, NY: Cornell University Press; 2004.

37. Sandler, T, Tschirhart, TJ, Cauley, J. A theoretical analysis of transnational terrorism. *Am Polit Sci Rev.* 1983; **77**: 36–54.

38. Wilson, MA. Toward a model of terrorist behavior in hostage-taking incidents. *J Conflict Resolut.* 2000; **44**: 403–424.

39. Schbley, AH. Torn between God, family, and money: the changing profile of Lebanon's religious terrorists. *Stud Confl Terror.* 2000; **23**: 175–196.

40. Persinger, MA. "I would kill in God's name": role of sex, weekly church attendance, report of a religious experience, and limbic lability. *Percept Mot Skills.* 1997; **85**(1): 128–130.

41. Milgram, S. *Obedience to Authority.* New York, NY: Harper Row; 1974.

42. Persinger, MA, Lafreniere, GF. *Space–Time Transients and Unusual Events.* Chicago, IL: Nelson Hall; 1977.

43. Taylor, M. *The Terrorist.* London: Brassey's; 1988.

44. Saver, JL, Rabin, J. The neural substrates of religious experience. *J Neuropsychiatry Clin Neurosci.* 1997; **9**(3): 498–510.

45. Devinsky, O, Lai, G. Spirituality and religion in epilepsy. *Epilepsy Behav.* 2008; **12** (4): 636–643.

46. Weatherston, D, Moran, J. Terrorism and mental illness: is there a relationship? *Int J Offender Ther Comp Criminol.* 2003; **47**(6): 698–713.

47. Marazziti, D. Is there a role for psychiatry in deepening our understanding of the "suicide bomber"? *Int J Psychiatry Clin Pract.* 2007; **11**(2): 87–89.

48. Salvatori, S. *Morire per Uccidere.* Udine: Edizioni Segno; 2010.

49. Adinoff, B. Neurobiologic processes in drug reward and addiction. *Harv Rev Psychiatry.* 2004; **12**(6): 305–320.

50. Robins, RS, Post, JM. *Political Paranoia: The Psychopolitics of Hatred.* New Haven, CT: Yale University Press; 1997.

51. Damasio, AR, Tranel, D, Damasio, H. Individuals with sociopathic behavior caused by frontal damage fail to respond autonomically to social stimuli. *Behav Brain Res.* 1990; **41**(2): 81–94.

52. Haidt, J. The new synthesis in moral psychology. *Science.* 2007; **316**(5827): 998–1002.

53. Moll, J, de Oliveira-Souza, R, Eslinger, PJ. Morals and the human brain: a working model. *Neuroreport.* 2003; **14**(3): 299–305.

54. Sophocles. *Antigone* Cambridge Greek and Latin Classic. Cambridge: Cambridge University Press; 1999.

Psychopathology of Terrorists

Armando Piccinni, Donatella Marazziti,
and Antonello Veltri[1]

Introduction

Given the heterogeneity of terrorist behavior, there remains a lack of consensus even about the definition of "terrorism," so that more than a hundred different academic labels can be found in the literature.[1]

Generally, by taking into account common elements found in current definitions, terrorism can be considered as violence or the threat of violence against non-combatant populations in order to obtain a political, religious, or ideological goal, or to influence the target population and change their behavior through fear and intimidation.

Since even terrorist actors may be very heterogeneous, different typologies of terrorism can be categorized. State terrorism, for example, refers to acts of terrorism conducted by a nation against foreign targets or its own people (e.g., the bombing of Guernica, the gassing of Kurdish civilians during the closing days of the Iran–Iraq War). Conversely, sub-state terrorism is categorized by Post (2004)[2] as social revolutionary terrorism, right-wing terrorism, nationalist/separatist terrorism, religious extremist terrorism, and single-issue terrorism (e.g., animal rights), each of which appears to be associated with its own psychological dynamics.

The large number of theories regarding the causes of terrorism include a broad spectrum of sociological, psychological, and psychiatric approaches. However, they rarely have been based on scientific methods, such as the use of validated measures for psychological and psychiatric examination, comparisons with appropriate control subjects, or the use of appropriate statistical testing to validate hypotheses. The reasons for this are multiple and often easily understandable. First, as already mentioned, terrorism cannot be interpreted as a unitary behavior, so that every theory based on hypotheses trying to draw general outlines is drawn up using inconsistent assumptions. Second, terrorism research may require dangerous and expensive travel to politically unstable regions. Third, active terrorists are not likely to cooperate with psychological or psychiatric assessment. Fourth, authorities may deny access to incarcerated terrorists because of security and secretive concerns. The result is that the data derived from systematic investigations are severely limited.

Since the debate concerning the causal connection between mental illness and terrorism is still open, the aim of the present article is to critically summarize the main psychopathological hypotheses about the genesis of terrorist behavior. For this aim, published data in the Medline and PubMed databases were searched up to March of 2017 using the keywords "terrorism" and "terrorist," each individually matched with "psychiatry," "psychopathology," and "mental illness." Furthermore, a search for relevant articles, books, and chapters of books was conducted by examining the cited references of the retrieved publications. In particular, retrieved information was used to discuss the arguments about the personality and psychopathology of terrorists.

Personality of Terrorists

As regards theories that posit that terrorism may be due to a personality disorder, the first interesting reports were published in the 1970s and 1980s. In the United States, Hubbard (1971),[3] based on unstructured interviews, described a group of skyjackers as sexually shy and passive, with poor social skills and achievements, with deeply religious mothers and violent and alcoholic fathers. Some common typical characteristics were identified in a larger group of more than 900 Italian right-wing terrorists,[4] particularly ambivalence about authority, defective insight, emotional detachment from the consequences of their actions, uncertain sexual roles, magical thinking, low-level education, and destructiveness. In Germany, another study utilizing semistructured interviews[5] with 227 left-wing and 23 right-wing terrorists identified two patterns of personality traits: (1) an extroverted, stimulus-seeking, dependent pattern, and (2) a hostile, suspicious, and defensive one. However, none of these American, Italian, and German studies used control groups and/or validated psychological instruments. They did not suggest common personality traits in the three analyzed groups, and without control subjects they could not conclude that the identified characteristics distinguished terrorists from non-terrorists.

More recently, a study employing semistructured interviews with 35 incarcerated Middle Eastern extremists[6] revealed that most came from respected families who had supported their activism. They cited peer influence as the main reason for joining the terrorist group, and membership was described as something that fused individual identity with the group's collective identity and goals. Studying the biographies of 10 Muslims who had engaged in terrorist acts and without a formal method to confirm his psychiatric impressions, Sageman (2004)[7] found no evidence of pathological narcissistic or paranoid traits.

We can think that, though terrorists rarely exhibit personality disorders, they can be characterized by subthreshold psychological traits or may be influenced by identifiable social factors.[8] Actually, in the previous few decades, many sociological and psychological theories have been proposed about this topic, interpreting terroristic activity as an aggressive reaction to frustration and social oppression or the result of social learning through group influences (ideological indoctrination, repetitive training, and peer pressures).[9] However, most of these theories lack validation by controlled empirical studies and fail to explain why only a tiny minority of the millions who are exposed to the same social factors and show the same psychological traits join a terrorist group.

To summarize, as regards the psychological characteristics of terrorists, the available studies lack a scientific design and fail to identify the common or typical pathological personality traits of terrorists.

Psychopathology of Terrorists

The popular opinion that terrorists must be insane or psychopathic is still widespread. Many theories developed during the 1970s and 1980s hypothesized a connection between mental illness and terrorism, suggesting that prior psychopathology causes individuals to engage in terrorist acts. Parry (1976)[10] stated that most political terrorists are not normal but are insane or mentally disturbed. Pearce (1977)[11] claimed that their behavior may show some evidence of psychopathy, paranoia, or some other clinical psychiatric disorder. Other authors have focused on personality disorders, attributing to terrorists a remorseless personality type (psychopathy or sociopathy)[12] or defining them as outlaws and outcasts with the typical characteristics of psychopaths.[13,14]

However, there is little evidence in the literature for the hypothesized connection between prior psychopathology and terrorism. Moreover, very little controlled research has been carried out with an adequate psychiatric evaluation. On the basis of uncontrolled empirical studies on left-wing German militants, on members of the Algerian Front de Liberation Nationale, and on members of Hezbollah, terrorists exhibited no signs of psychiatric disorders.[15–17] In Northern Ireland, a clinical examination[18] comparing 59 ordinary killers with 47 political murderers found that the latter were generally more stable, had a better family background, and showed significantly less evidence of mental illness. Rash (1979)[19] examined 11 members of the German Baader–Meinhof terrorist group and reported no evidence of mental illness in any of the respondents. Post et al. (2003)[6] also found no psychiatric disorders in two groups of 21 and 14 Islamist terrorists. Therefore, many authors have concluded that, if it is true that the leaders of terrorist groups are sometimes insane individuals and that a few terrorist acts may be attributed to insane persons, terrorists rarely meet the psychiatric criteria for mental disorders.[20,21]

Similarly, several lines of reasoning do not support the popular claim that antisocial behavior is typical or common among terrorists. Extensive evidence favors the notion that terrorists are far from being outcasts. On the contrary, they are often considered by their groups as heroes fighting for the freedom of their people. The Irishman who joined the Provisional Irish Republican Army or the Middle Eastern student who joins an Islamist radical group may receive considerable popular support, and they think of themselves as being altruistic and to be contributing to the best of his/her society, even as significantly increasing the economic income of his/her family.[17,22] Ironically, therefore, with respect to group identities, certain types of terrorism represent "prosocial" behavior—the antithesis of selfishness. Further evidence of the prosociality of some terrorists derives from an Italian study on militants who joined a terrorist organization.[23] The author suggested that terrorist recruitment begins by involving the militant in a group with shared social values, by filling the individual's sense of emptiness and eliminating their sense of exclusion, and by promoting a "role" within the society where he/she was considered to be a dropout.

Another interesting point of view considers the possibility that terrorism and mental illness may be connected because of the effects produced in some individuals by their engaging in terrorist activities—that is to say, that psychopathology is the consequence of surrounding conditions and events.[24] Therefore, if the presence of mental disorders is detected in a terrorist, it cannot necessarily be concluded that the disorder was the cause rather than the consequence of terrorist activity. Trauma- and stressor-related disorders (e.g., posttraumatic stress disorder and adjustment disorders) are conditions specifically linked to intense stressors, like combatants' exposure to life-threatening and catastrophic events.[25] Along these lines, different variables have been proposed that may be of importance in contributing to psychiatric disorders secondary to terrorist acts, particularly terrorists' lifestyles, the need to hide themselves, abandonment of original families, frequent and sudden escapes, living in extreme situations, adhesion to the strict rules of the group, conflicts within the group, and the effects of interrogation and incarceration.[24]

To summarize, there is no significant evidence in available literature of a link between psychopathology and terrorism. As with general criminal activity, there are undoubtedly cases where individuals engage in terrorism because of a prior mental disorder (the so-called "lone wolves," although the latest isolated acts carried out by this kind of individual do not support this assumption), but this possibility is most likely remote. Therefore, without doubt, it is a hard task to try and disentangle the question of how great might be the impact of a preexisting mental disorder on a terrorist, or if, when clearly diagnosed, it is the cause rather than the effect of his/her behavior.

Conclusions and Perspectives

No evidence exists that terrorist behavior is caused by either prior psychiatric disorders or psychopathy. Many theories have proposed social factors and psychological traits as predisposing elements for terrorist acts, but they almost always lack empirical validation. In any case, terrorists are markedly psychologically heterogeneous, and every terrorist, like every person, has his/her own complex of psychosocial experiences and traits. As Victoroff (2005)[9] argued, terrorism is unequivocally a subtype of human aggression that is probably always determined by a combination of innate factors, biological factors, early developmental factors, cognitive factors, temperament, environmental influences, and group dynamics. The degree to which each of these factors contributes to a given event probably varies between individual terrorists and between terrorist groups. Theories that claim predominance for one of these influences over the others are at the moment premature. Systematic and scientific investigations are needed in order to understand the bases of terrorist aggression and to design an appropriate counterterrorism policy. Taking into account the most recent and increasingly tragic attacks, it should be imperative to institute multidisciplinary research programs in order to increase a critical knowledge base founded on evidence and not on theoretical presumptions. The best therapy in medicine, as well as in psychiatry, is prevention. An effective counterterrorism policy, therefore, should be guided by a scientific understanding of the individual and societal/environmental risk factors that might predispose individuals to become terrorists.

Disclosures

The authors do not have any disclosures, and the authors do not have any affiliation with or financial interest in any organization that might pose a conflict of interest.

References

1. Schmid, A. *Political Terrorism: A Research Guide to the Concepts, Theories, Databases and Literature*, with a bibliography by the author and a world directory of "terrorist" organizations by A.J. Jongman. Amsterdam: North Holland; 1983.

2. Post, JM. *Leaders and Their Followers in a Dangerous World: The Psychology of Political Behavior*. Ithaca, NY: Cornell University Press; 2004.

3. Hubbard, DG. *The Skyjacker: His Flights of Fantasy*. New York, NY: Macmillan; 1971.

4. Ferracuti, F, Bruno, F. Psychiatric aspects of terrorism in Italy. In: Barak-Glantz IL, Huff CR, eds. *The Mad, the Bad and the Different: Essays in Honor of Simon Dinitz*. Lexington, MA: Lexington Books; 1981: 199–213.

5. Crenshaw, M. The psychology of political terrorism. In: Hermann MG, ed. *Political Psychology*. San Francisco, CA: Jossey-Bass; 1986: 379–413.

6. Post, JM, Sprinzak, E, Denny, LM. The terrorists in their own words: interviews with thirty-five incarcerated Middle Eastern terrorists. *Terror Polit Violence*. 2003; **15**: 171–184.

7. Sageman, M. *Understanding Terror Networks*. Philadelphia, PA: University of Pennsylvania Press; 2004.

8. Marazziti, D. Psychiatry and terrorism: exploring the unacceptable. *CNS Spectr*. 2016; **21**(2): 128–130.

9. Victoroff, J. The mind of the terrorist. *J Conflict Resolut*. 2005; **49**(1): 3–42.

10. Parry, A. *Terrorism: From Robespierre to Arafat*. New York, NY: Vanguard Press; 1976.

11. Pearce, KI. Police negotiations. *Can Psychiatr Assoc J*. 1977; **22**(4): 171–174.

12. Taylor, M. *The Terrorist*. London: Brassey's; 1988.

13. Cooper, HHA. What is a terrorist: a psychological perspective. *Leg Med Q*. 1977; **1**: 16–32.

14. Cooper, HHA. Psychopath as terrorist: a psychological perspective. *Leg Med Q*. 1978; **2**: 253–262.

15. Jäger, H, Schmidtchen, G, Süllwold, L. *Analyzen zum Terrorismus 2: Lebenslaufanalysen*. Darmstadt, Germany: Deutscher Verlag; 1981.

16. Crenshaw, M. The causes of terrorism. *Comp Polit*. 1981; **13**(4): 379–399.

17. Merari, A. The readiness to kill and die: suicidal terrorism in the Middle East. In: Reich W, ed. *Origins of Terrorism: Psychologies, Ideologies, Theologies, States of Mind*. Washington, DC: Woodrow Wilson Center Press; 1998: 192–207.

18. Lyons, H, Harbinson, H. A comparison of political and non-political murderers in Northern Ireland, 1974–1984. *Med Sci Law*. 1986; **26**(3): 193–198.

19. Rasch, W. Psychological dimensions of political terrorism in the Federal Republic of Germany. *Int J Law Psychiatry*. 1979; **2**(1): 79–85.

20. Ferracuti, F. A sociopsychiatric interpretation of terrorism. *Ann Am Acad Polit Soc Sci*. 1982; **463**: 129–140.

21. Silke, AP. Cheshire-cat logic: the recurring theme of terrorist abnormality in psychological research. *Psychol Crime Law*. 1998; **4**: 51–69.

22. Heskin, K. The psychology of terrorism in Ireland. In: Alexander Y, O'Day A, eds. *Terrorism in Ireland*. New York, NY: St. Martin's; 1984: 88–105.

23. Della Porta, D. Recruitment processes in clandestine political organizations: Italian left-wing terrorism. *Int Soc Mov Res*. 1988; **1**: 155–169.

24. Weatherston, D, Moran, J. Terrorism and mental illness: is there a relationship? *Int J Offender Ther Comp Criminol*. 2003; **47**(6): 698–713.

25. American Psychiatric Association. *Diagnostic and Statistical Manual of Mental Disorders*, 5th ed. Arlington, VA: American Psychiatric Publishing; 2013.

Chapter 6

Why is Terrorism a Man's Business?

Anne Maria Möller-Leimkühler

Terrorism–Some Principal Aspects

Terrorism is a highly contested concept. It includes numerous different national, academic, and political definitions; however, for decades a legal definition was missing. A first consensus has recently been achieved by the General Assembly of the United Nations:

> Terrorism refers, on the one hand, to a doctrine about the presumed effectiveness of a special form or tactic of fear-generating, coercive political violence and, on the other hand, to a conspiratorial practice of calculated, demonstrative, direct violent action without legal or moral restraints, targeting mainly civilians and non-combatants, performed for its propagandistic and psychological effects on various audiences and conflict parties.[1]

The doctrine may be based on fundamentalist political or religious ideologies that legitimize all kinds of violence. For example, Islamist extremism names all non-Muslims and even liberal Muslims as infidels, who must be killed until there is no other religion left but the "true faith."

Terrorism as coercive political violence may be employed by illegal state repression or by nonstate actors; the latter may act in small groups or diffuse transnational networks, but increasingly also as single actors ("lone-wolf" terrorism). This has been described as the changing face of terrorism in the twenty-first century.[2] Lone-wolf attackers are meanwhile the main perpetrators of terrorist activity in Western societies, mainly in the US, but recently also in France and Germany, causing 70 per cent of all deaths caused by terrorists over the past 10 years. Half of all attacks worldwide with a connection to the so-called Islamic State (also known as ISIS or ISIL) have been conducted by lone actors.[3] However, Islamic fundamentalism is not the main driver of terrorism in Western countries; lone-wolf terrorists also have been inspired by political extremism, nationalism, and racial and religious supremacy (e.g., the case of far-right terrorist Anders Behring Breivik, who committed the 2011 Norway attacks and killed 77 persons).

The direct victims of terror attacks are not the ultimate target but serve as message generators: the attack is documented by online social media platforms and mass media, which further reinforces the terrorists' focus on public attention, public fear, and intimidation, as well as effects of propaganda for their message and recruitment of potential terrorists. For instance, online publishing of filmed beheadings by Al Qaeda have been intended to serve as a display of power and enactment. Similarly, the World Trade Center assault in New York on September 11, 2001, can be considered as a perverse performance of omnipotence and the power to cause chaos, confusion, and fear, not primarily to legitimize a political ideology.[4]

Terrorism is a highly complex phenomenon shaped by political and socioeconomic conditions, as well as by ethnic and ideological conflicts and their history, demographic characteristics, regional segregation, and access to weapons.

There are 2 distinct sets of factors associated with terrorism depending on the developmental status of the country. Between 1989 and 2014, 93 per cent of all terrorist attacks occurred in countries with high levels of state-sponsored terror.[3] Depending on the level of development, factors such as youth unemployment, militarization, levels of criminality, or distrust in the electoral process can be statistically identified as correlates of terrorism in Organisation for Economic Co-operation and Development (OECD)-affiliated countries. In developing countries, factors such as the history of conflict, levels of corruption, acceptance of the human rights, and group-based inequalities are more significantly related to terrorist activity.[3] As measured by the Global Terrorism Index, countries with the highest rate of terrorism are Iraq, Afghanistan, Nigeria, Pakistan, and Syria. The most active and global terror groups are ISIL (Islamic State of Iraq and the Levant), Boko Haram, the Taliban, and Al Qaeda.

Especially since 2014, increased Islamist terrorist activity in Europe can be observed. This increase can be related to spill-over effects of the Syrian Civil War, to the so-called "Iraq effect" caused by the US war under President Bush against Iraq,[5] and to the European continuing migrant crisis, which facilitates the infiltration of terrorists. As one consequence of the upsurge of ISIS/ISIL and of millions of incoming refugees, there is a rise not only of anti-Muslim attitudes in Europe,[6] but also an increase of anti-immigration and Islamophobic violence as well as militant, right-wing extremist groups. The upsurge of ISIL is further due to the fact that it has successfully begun to use Europe as a new recruitment base for potential terrorists, even though it has lost ground in the Middle East.

In fact, from 2012 to 2015, more than 400 people left Belgium for ISIL-controlled Iraq and Syria, and nearly 1,200 left France to join jihad terrorism.[7] The European Police Agency Europol estimates that more than 5,000 Europeans have left to join Islamist fighters in Syria, and the problem for security services is aggravated when these people return with training and a mission.[8] In Germany, for example, 550 potentially violent attackers have been identified.

When estimating the current terrorist threat in Western societies, Renard[8] states "that it is very serious, even increasing, but not existential" (p. 7). Statistically, people would have a higher chance of dying from a car accident, or falling off their bed or a ladder than dying from terrorism.

Terrorism Is a Man's Business

As is obvious from the introduction, violence is a multicausal behavior and has been subject to various disciplines with a variety of somewhat controversial theories. However, a fact more than apparent is that physical violence, whether it is individual or collective, such as wars, armed conflicts, genocides, or terrorism, is a predominantly male phenomenon. Generally and throughout history, young males have been the main protagonists of criminal as well as political violence. However, gender is widely ignored in terrorism and violence research. Where it is addressed, it refers mainly to women, not to men, because the latter are held to be the "norm" of violent behavior, so self-evident that further explanation is not needed. This article focuses on violent young males from different perspectives. What makes men violent? A comprehensive approach to better understand this phenomenon includes neurobiological, psychological, and social factors that increase the risk of violence under certain societal conditions. These factors will also contribute to the question of why especially young males become radicalized and why they are prone to violent extremist groups.

Neurobiological Predispositions for Male Violence

Gender is an issue of nature and nurture. Maleness, respectively, masculinity is not solely a socio-cultural construct, as many social scientists still believe, but is also shaped by sex differences in brain structure and function, stress response, and genetics. That does not mean that males are "hardwired" for violence, but it does mean that they may be more disposed to aggression and violence than females.[9,10] Numerous examples of sex differences in the brain, in brain regions and circuits, have been documented that are relevant regarding violent behavior. In addition, a mutation of monoamine oxidase A (MAOA), a gene encoding enzyme responsible for the breakdown of the neurotransmitters norepinephrine, serotonin, and dopamine, has been proven that makes affected males more disposed to antisocial and violent behavior, especially when they had experienced maltreatment or neglect in their childhood.[9,11] With regard to brain structure, the volume of the male amygdala (center of emotion processing) is larger compared to that of females, whereas the orbitofrontal cortex, which controls negative emotions emerging from the amygdala, is smaller. As brain researchers conclude, males may be less able to regulate negative emotions and so may be more prone to impulsive behavior.[12] With respect to neurotransmitters, data indicate that low levels of serotonin may reinforce aggressiveness, impulsivity, and risk-taking behavior in males, especially in stressful situations.[13–15] While women under stress may be protected by estrogen and oxytocin, and may respond with prosocial strategies such as communication and help-seeking, men tend to respond with a higher release of cortisol and testosterone, which is associated with the fight or flight response, particularly when they feel threatened in their social status.[16] Unlike in animal studies, testosterone in human males may not be directly associated with physical aggression, but rather with social dominance. Males with high testosterone, when viewing angry faces, display less activation of the amygdala than those with low testosterone, which indicates that they feel less threatened by the anger of others.[17] Furthermore, an association with delinquent and violent behavior has been found in late adolescent males.[12] Specifically in their early adolescence, males are experiencing an excessive rise of testosterone, driving them to aggressive, risk-taking behavior and sensation-seeking, which is significantly reinforced by peers.[18] Risky behavior in adolescents seems also to be triggered by a specific heightened sensitivity of the dopaminergic reward system ("no risk, no fun"). However, risky behavior does not guarantee rewards, but may as well have negative outcomes, the worst of which is increased mortality due to suicides, traffic accidents, unintentional self-injuries, and violence.[19] This is partly due to an imbalance of brain maturing in adolescent males, with the orbitofrontal cortex maturing later and more slowly (about 2 years later compared to females), while the amygdala/the limbic regions develop earlier and more quickly, probably impacting rational or moral decision making.[20]

With highly professional media marketing strategies, explicitly focusing on heroism and adventure (similar to Hollywood scripts[21,22]), ISIL is targeting mainly adolescent males, whose identity is typically fragile and malleable in their teenage years. Longing for purpose and adventure, young males may be particularly susceptible to ISIL's promises (money, guns, and girls). In addition, throughout history rebellion against the establishment (family, school, state, church) has always been a strong motivator in young males.

Recently it has been reported that even underaged and unaccompanied boys who are caught up in refugee camps in Germany are the new target of radical Salafists (an ultra-conservative movement within Sunni Islam).[23] These traumatized, vulnerable children undergoing indoctrination are extremely susceptible to brain damage, as basic social, emotional, and cognitive neuronal networks are laid down in childhood.

Masculinity and Violence

Maleness is not only based on biology, but also on socio-historical construc-
tions of what it means to be male, which may be different in different cultures
(and subcultures) and different times. However, in most societies, hegemonic
masculinity[24] has established patriarchal gender hierarchies. The traditional
ideal of masculinity, stereotypically associated with action, dominance, achievement, power, competition, autonomy, pain tolerance, endurance, and indepen-
dence, has been challenged currently, especially by younger generations.
However, (adolescent) males may cope with an insecure identity, feelings of
emasculization, inter- or intragender competition, grievances or experiences of
social disintegration, and anxiety or hopelessness by subscribing to exaggerated
traditional masculinity norms. One of the most influential archetypes of heroic
masculinity is the fighter (others are the breadwinner or the rebel), e.g., the
superhero as presented in computer games and films, or the man-of-action
hero, a specifically American ideal, which may manifest itself in symbolic
everyday consumption, when opportunities to gain and demonstrate power
and status have been reduced in our postindustrial times.[25]

Aggression and violence are basic components of these masculinity ideals,
and are legitimized as they aid in building and rebuilding social order (as is
also supported by evolutionary explanations). For this reason, aggression and
violence are at the same time principle means to demonstrate and reconstruct
masculinity.

In the face of numerous rites of passage from boyhood to manhood in
many preindustrial countries, theorists of various disciplines suppose that
unlike womanhood, manhood is a precarious social status because it is relatively difficult to earn, but easy to lose. It is not a state of being, but rather
a status that is conferred by others, particularly other males.[26] Becoming and
remaining a "real man" entails suffering, proving, and fighting for social
acceptance. Male identity seems particularly precarious in individuals with
a high mental vulnerability due to experiencing stress in childhood, such as
family violence, broken home, absence of the father, abuse, or other trauma-
tization. Masculinity is a status that is earned and maintained primarily by
actions and achievements, not so much by enduring personal attributes.[27]
Thus, risk-taking physical behavior, including aggression and violence, is
perceived as a way for males to demonstrate masculinity, particularly when
it has been threatened.

Extremists, whether they are right-wing extremists or Islamic extremists,
share the perception that the world is perishing because their fundamentalist
political/religious values are threatened by dominating Western ideologies of
democracy, gender equality, and open society. Thus, it is not astonishing that
these ideologies are linked to ultraconservative ideals of masculinity, as

demonstrated in their propaganda, messages, and symbols. These ideals play an important part in young males' search for identity, leading them to believe that joining right-wing extremists would be a masculine rite of passage.[28] Masculinity becomes a kind of hypermasculinity that includes a narrowly defined, exaggerated, and violence-oriented image of the warrior.[28] Thus, young men have to prove their maleness in violent acts, with violence and combat as the only medium available where real masculinity can be acquired and verified.

This notion of hypermasculinity refers to the broader historical link between masculinity and the military, which has been constructed for the purpose of waging wars and is well documented, e.g., by militarized masculinity in World Wars I and II. By equating military requirements with male values such as toughness, courage, honor, and willpower, violence becomes legitimized, normalized, and even glamorized, and thus is transferred into the self-concept. This instrumentalization of a unidimensional construct of masculinity, together with the Nazi ideology and visions of "Great Germany," might be one explanation for the ruthless violence conducted by German soldiers. Narratives of German soldiers who fought in World Wars I or II[29] illustrate how intensely soldiers had internalized those expectations of hardness and ruthlessness to prove their masculinity and to avoid being emasculated for showing empathy for the enemy. The stronger their adaptation to martial masculinity, the better they were able to suppress their emotions, fears, scruples, and suffering. There is also evidence from secret recordings of conversations made by the British intelligence on German prisoners of war that some soldiers might have even enjoyed their killing and atrocities towards civilians; at the very least, some boasted about their actions.[30] Militarized masculinity is one important cornerstone, not only for the war machinery, but also for the soldiers' experiences, their social roles, and their coping strategies. It might be seen as a complex defense mechanism in order to protect the self from traumatic experiences, and possibly as a (dysfunctional) way to cope with guilt.

Even today the soldier/warrior remains a key symbol of masculinity,[31] and militarized masculinity remains central to the perpetuation of violence in international relations.[32]

Coming back to Islamic terrorism, the fighter is simultaneously the sacred warrior who dies a martyr and is declared a hero both before and after his death. Monetary awards and support provided to the families of suicide bombers and other martyrs serves to reinforce the value and glamor of these extremely violent acts.[33] Due to the fact that Islamic culture is a culture of honor, manhood and honor are closely related; they are even synonymous.[34] Men are also viewed as owners and protectors of the women's honor in their families. They must protect their reputations and those of their families, even with violence when necessary, because dishonor means shame and emasculation. Thus, in cultures of honor, masculinity is even more precarious with perceived insults evoking aggression and violent behavior to restore manhood. In Islamic extremism, male honor can be only found in the role as warrior whereas female honor is found in the home.

Taken together, right-wing and Islamic extremism/terrorism are based on common notions of archaic masculinity, which are perceived to be threatened and may result in terroristic actions to restore culture and manhood.

To give an individual example, an alternative view of the right-wing terrorist Anders Behring Breivik, who committed the 2011 Norway attacks and killed 77 young people, may demonstrate the driving forces of his bombing and shooting on the island Utoya: perceived Islamification, perceived breakdown of male dominance, and sexual liberation.[35] Based on his analyses of the key documents of the case, Richards has supposed that Breivik's (unconscious) core fear was emasculation, an attack on his masculine identity arising from changes in society. "In this polemic, the fusion of feminism, feminization, matriarchy, androgyny and homosexuality threatens to engulf the Christian European heterosexual male, the hero of history who is now an object of contempt and hatred. It is here that Breivik's choice of Utoya as his target can be understood" (p. 45).[35] Breivik's fantasies focused on re-establishing the medieval military order of the Knights Templar with grandiose ideas of omnipotence and restoration. According to Richards, "Breivik arrived at the island in a homemade police uniform to put an end to their sexual free-for-all, and to reassert the heroic figure of the patriarchal male who offers exemplary resistance to the tide of soft, corrupting pleasure that is washing over his civilization and dissolving its core categories" (p. 45).[35]

Youth Bulges, Economic Stagnation, and Terrorism

Some years ago, the cover of the German weekly magazine *Der Spiegel* declared in large type: "Young men: The world's most dangerous species."[36] Of course this is an inadequate generalization. Although violent crimes and terrorist attacks are mostly committed by young males aged between 15 and 25, violence is a rather rare event on the individual level: in Germany, for example, about 2 per cent of young men of this age are suspected to have committed one or more violent crimes.[37] But what about disproportional cohorts of adolescent males who live mainly in Islamic countries and become involved in terrorism? What makes young men susceptible to violence and terrorism from a macro-level perspective? As the link between terrorism, types of terrorism, and social/societal conditions in different countries is extremely complex, it is not possible to identify common causes to explain terrorism as a general phenomenon.[38] However, regarding the evolution of Islamic terrorism in developing countries, several main causes have been described: centuries of colonization, weakness of the state, political exclusion and social inequality, economic stagnation or decline, and negative effects of globalization. These factors are often cumulative and interacting, so that any mobilization for a peaceful change seems rather impossible.[39] Thus, poverty and humiliation play important roles, but are not single causes of terrorism, as often has been argued. What has been also discussed is the question of whether the demographic explosion of so-called youth bulges, defined as large cohorts of young males aged 15–24 relative to the total adult population (over 20 per cent), are a breeding ground for violence and terrorism.[40] Given a declining or stagnating economy in numerous Muslim societies (e.g., Middle East, Africa, parts of Asia) with high rates of unemployment, many young men, mostly born after 1980, lacking the perspective that comes with age but with a lot of free time, feel humiliated and marginalized without any opportunities to prove themselves as honorable and masculine in culturally prescribed ways.[41] Empirical evidence suggests an association between youth bulges and increased risk for political or terrorist violence, especially when economic opportunities are reduced and levels of education are low, but also in cases when highly educated young males do not find adequate jobs. It is not by chance that young engineers are overrepresented among Islamic terrorists in the Muslim countries, as Gambetta and Hertog[42] found in their study on the correlation between extremism and education in Muslim countries. In their analysis of data regarding 497 members of extremist groups, they concluded that, aside from a specific mind-set typical for engineers the main reason for joining a terrorist group is experiencing frustrated expectations and relative deprivation: engineering is one of the most prestigious subjects, with high entry requirements in Muslim countries, thus young students expect corresponding high-status employment after graduation. However, because of economic development failures in North Africa and the Middle East, such high-status opportunities are extremely rare. These young engineers thus experience a large dissonance between merit and reward, which contributes to their radicalization. Interestingly, Gambetta and Hertog[42] did not find an overrepresentation of engineers among terrorists in the West, in Singapore, or in Saudi Arabia, where graduates have far better professional opportunities. (In these areas Islamic terrorism has attracted more marginal males with lower education.)

To conclude, it is not that relatively large cohorts of young males are dangerous per se, but they may become dangerous under the conditions of low, respectfully, expanding education and concurrent economic stagnation, which restrain "doing" masculinity within cultural standards and gaining social acceptance. If such opportunities do not exist, political or religious violence, whether individual or collective, may serve as a powerful alternative for living without "male" achievements. Thus, most vulnerable to terrorist agitation are well-educated young men who are frustrated about the lack of opportunities in the developing countries in which they live.[43]

Another picture emerges, for example, in East Germany, where another bulge of young men comprises a new lower class in remote regions. Despite the reunification of West and East Germany in 1989, the eastern regions have remained less developed economically, with higher rates of unemployment, especially among young males. While many better educated young women left for West Germany to improve their career options, young men, particularly from rural areas, remained in their home regions. For these young men, who are less educated and are unemployed, migrating to West Germany to find better jobs is not a realistic option. Also, due to the migration of young women, finding a mate and starting a family are difficult for young males, as in some regions the population of females aged 18–34 is down by 25 per cent.[44] Economic restructuring, lack of education, and lack of adaptation have contributed not only to increasing violent criminality among males, but also to the rising attraction of far-right extremist groups that celebrate hypermasculine, anti-feminist, anti-democratic, and racist ideologies. One of the reasons may be that young men perceive a profound devaluation of the traditional male gender role, including physical labor and breadwinning, because traditional male jobs in crafts, manufacturing, and construction (not requiring better education and being highly respected in the former German Democratic Republic) now have been severely affected by structural change of the economy and have lost importance.[45] Given that many young men are poorly educated, have low income or are unemployed, and are without opportunity to start a family, they feel disadvantaged and emasculated, and may long for a revaluation of "genuine" masculinity.

Not surprisingly, the number of right-wing extremists in Germany has increased from 21,000 in 2014 to 22,600 in 2016, with half of them being regarded as violence oriented.[46] Respectively, there has been a continuous and dramatic increase of right-wing extremist violence in the last few years. From 2014 to 2015, the number of violent offenses increased by 44 per cent, and refugee shelters were the predominant target (901 violent attacks out of 1,005 total attacks).

Group Dynamics and Identity Fusion

There is a consensus among terrorist experts that psychological explanations of terrorism at the individual level are not sufficient. In order to best explain terrorist behavior, group psychology must be applied, with a particular focus on collective identity. This is all the more important because a unique psychopathological, psychological, or social profile for terrorists could not be derived from biographical analyses.[2,47,48]

Male alliances have always been the dominant unit in competitive public arenas, such as science, economy, sports, religion, secret societies, police, military, and politics—in particular political violence. Terrorists operate conventionally in groups/organizations; mentally unstable individuals are screened out, because they represent a security risk.[2] Generally, 90 per cent of all violent attacks by young males are performed in groups. This is because violence is a constitutive component in aggression-prone groups, which render putative status and power to the individual member. Furthermore, male groups are functional for males in general, as they are the key sites where masculinity is defined, proved, performed, and reconstructed.[49]

Searching for the roots of group violence, evolutionary theory suggests that living in groups is beneficial for the survival of certain species (humans, primates, or rats), especially under conditions of limited resources (food, territory), which are embattled by rival male subgroups. Discriminating, attacking, casting out, or killing individuals belonging to the same species, but not to the same group, seems to be a phylogenetic heritage, as has been manifested in countless wars and battles, as well as numerous genocides, throughout history. This phenomenon has been referred to by social psychology as intergroup conflict or minimal group paradigm.[50] It is based on a profound evolutionary pattern of belonging to one group and separating from others with regard to differences such as ethnic, religious, linguistic, cultural, or national. As Tajfel[51] has demonstrated in experimental studies, separation into groups can occur even on minimal, arbitrary, and meaningless differences that trigger intergroup discrimination; identity with a group is based solely on group membership, a kind of social categorization. On the individual level, being part of a group (e.g., genetic, cultural, ideological) and identifying with the group's goals, values, and norms constitute a sense of social identity, pride, and self-esteem. Overvaluing the own group ("we") and devaluating the out-group ("they") results in an increased self-image of the group members and subsequently an increased group cohesiveness. Social identity theory states that the more strongly a member identifies with the group, the stronger his social identity will be, but the more his personal identity will fade. He will become a puppet. However, this idea generates new questions. Are puppets able to sacrifice themselves for their group? Were the soldiers of the Nazi regime puppets without personal identity? It is possible that extreme pro-group behavior, like suicide bombing or mass murder, may not be fully explained by this approach.

Based on social identity theory, a more sophisticated explanation has been developed by Swann et al.,[52,53] who put forward the concept of "identity fusion." Identity fusion occurs in different degrees due to a visceral feeling of oneness with the group, while personal identity is retained and channeled into pro-group action. In addition to the synergetic connection of personal and collective identity, the perception of the group as a family is crucial for motivation. Highly fused group members cultivate close ties to other group members, as well as to the group as a whole. Thus, it is not surprising that actors whose personal identity is highly fused within a unique collective identity would kill and die for the sake of their collective when it is threatened, because they perceive the bonds as family-like. In-depth case and field studies of terrorist groups by the anthropologist Scott Atran[54,55] suggest that "people almost never kill and die (just) for the cause, but for each other: for their group, whose cause makes their imagined family of genetic strangers—their brotherhood, fatherland, motherland, homeland" (p. 33).[54]

Due to the dangers and costs of participation in terrorism, terrorist groups are more tight-knit than other voluntary associations. Obviously, this may be one of the most attractive factors for potential terrorists. There is evidence from interviews with terrorists that many join violent groups seeking challenges and excitement, but above all they seek friendship and fellowship. These motives seem more important to them than the political purpose or ideology of their collective.[5]

Such non-ideological motivations are also supported for right-wing extremists.[56–58] From a perspective of social disintegration,[59] right-wing violence among young males can best be explained as a consequence of deficits in fundamental recognition needs. It is a sort of projective coping of individual deficits perceived as being caused by others. Ideology often serves as a justification of violent acts.

Lone-Wolf Terrorists Are Different

Lone-wolf terrorists prepare and commit violent acts alone, without command structure or material assistance from terrorist groups/organizations. Nevertheless, they may be influenced or motivated by terrorist groups, and may act in support of these groups. Although lone-wolf terrorism is rare, it has been a historical, and now increasing, phenomenon in the US and Europe, being inspired not only by ISIL but also by far-right extremism. It is argued that the surge of lone-wolf terrorism is due to pressure from security services forcing a tactical adaptation, and terrorist groups, particularly ISIL, who call on those who share their ideology to act alone without direction or support.[60] The Internet has made it easier than ever before to distribute and find radicalizing material and instructions on how to conduct attacks.[61] The profile of lone actors has proven to be rather heterogeneous, while the only common factor is being male.[62] Political or religious ideology seems not to be the only motivation for their attacks, but personal grievances also contribute. Current research on lone actor terrorists indicates that they differ significantly from members of terrorist groups; they seem to have much more in common with apolitical mass murderers or school shooters,[63] as they tend to combine their personal grievances and frustrations with religious or political ideologies.[64] This is a commonality that distinguishes lone actors from organized terrorists who share collective grievances. However, because of the complex constellation of contributing factors in each case, it is not possible to identify a unique psychological profile of the typical lone-wolf terrorist. Decades of research have attempted to find such unique explanations,[65] starting with psychopathological approaches in the 1970s (mostly speculations based on anecdotal observations) followed by psychoanalytic approaches during the 1980s, with particular emphasis on narcissism. In the 1990s and 2000s, these approaches have been dismissed due to methodological and empirical reasons, while group dynamics, based on improved data collection and primary interviews with terrorists, became the new dominating concept to understand terrorist motivation in general. However, in the face of increasing lone-wolf terrorism, group dynamics cannot be a sufficient explanation, even though lone attackers may have self-radicalized via Internet propaganda of terrorist groups and may perceive themselves as members of a virtual community. Consequently, previously dismissed mental health and personality factors must be revisited on the basis of the existing empirical evidence, while extreme positions must be questioned ("they are all mentally ill" or "a terrorist cannot be mentally ill"[65]). For example, with respect to mental illness, it has often been argued that mental illness is the primary reason for violent behavior, and that a mentally ill person is not able to rationally plan violent attacks. However, it has been shown that lone-actor terrorists diagnosed with mental illness frequently display rational motivations[65] and are capable of sophisticated attack planning.[66] In fact, mental health problems are significantly more common in lone-actor terrorists compared to group-based terrorists.[67,68] Corner and Gill[67] also support the role of social isolation in lone actors, as they found that 53 per cent of lone actors were socially isolated; however, this isolation was due to a recent interpersonal conflict rather than a chronic state. Other authors emphasize that, while lone wolves physically isolate themselves from society, they simultaneously seek recognition for their causes through spoken statements and threats, manifestos, e-mail messages, texting, and videotaped proclamations.[64]

As quantitative and qualitative analyses of lone-actor terrorists indicate, unsolved psychosocial problems may play an important role in self-radicalizing and conducting terroristic attacks, as is also true for school shooters. Both lone actors and school shooters perceive themselves as outsiders and are unable to accept defeat or to cope with cumulative disappointment, and so they end up in a state of chronic frustration and aggression.[69,70]

Some sociologists have claimed that searching for reasons and contributing factors to explain violence and terror would legitimize and victimize the perpetrators while ignoring their main motivation: experiencing total power over their victims, feeling omnipotent, and being a hero and avenger. However, this is no contradiction. Whether lone-actor terrorist, school shooter, or group-related terrorist, they belong to the "laughing killer" type.[71] According to Theweleit, "they are men who enjoy their murderous game, who see themselves as part of a higher power that condones all of this.

They laugh as they celebrate the sanctioned crime, their unpunished, godlike actions."[72] Anders Breivik, the Norwegian mass murderer, burst into ecstatic laughter during his killing spree, and was relaxed and smiling during the trial. Others did likewise: the killers in Orlando, when he shot in the head his wounded victims next to him, the killers in Dallas, in Charleston, North Carolina, or in Bataclan, Paris, who apparently enjoyed their atrocities.

With respect to sociodemographic characteristics of lone shooters, the existing literature indicates no consistent evidence of economic disadvantage or poorer education compared to the general population, but points to a higher rate of unemployment.[62] Obviously, there seem to be differences depending on the different ideologies. Compared to Islamist lone actor terrorists, right-wing lone actors have a lower education, and are often unemployed, single, and have never been married.

In sum, sociodemographic data at best demonstrate the variability of terrorists' backgrounds. In the words of Adam Deen, an ex-Jihadi and now counter-terrorist outreach worker in London: "The predominant factor in radicalisation is the ideology [of Islam]—it is the ideas that move people. I didn't come from a poverty-stricken background or broken home. I went to university, I didn't feel angry and I was apolitical. Yet, I was indoctrinated with a radical Islamist ideology and became impassioned with the idea of an Islamic state."[73]

Conclusions

In the face of the multiple factors likely associated with terrorism, it is obvious that there exists no unique "master explanation." Research can only offer approaches to understanding terrorism from a variety of perspectives, thus producing even more complexity.

Nevertheless, clear answers are needed for many reasons, not the least of which is practical approaches to counterterrorism. Thus, in political and public debates, different explanations regarding root causes (necessary and sufficient causes) have been favored. One popular "master explanation" has been humiliation, as Islamist terrorists themselves, and also terrorism experts, have claimed humiliation to be a motivating force. According to the historian Goldhagen,[74] there are, however, many historical examples in non-Middle Eastern countries where humiliation did not result in devastating terror. This means that there is no deterministic link between humiliation and terror on the macro-social level, just as there is no deterministic link between frustration and aggression/violence on the micro-social level, as was supposed by early aggression theory. Of course, real or perceived humiliation and frustration are playing important roles, but what significantly triggers violence in this context is the connection with fundamentalist political-religious ideas of a better world that shape political goals and result in destructive power politics and terror. This is a continuous pattern throughout history and may reflect an anthropological matter of fact. Numerous historical examples show how men and unidimensional notions of masculinity have been instrumentalized for political violence by propagating individual significance as a hero, avenger, or warrior in the name of God or for any goal greater than oneself. From a gender perspective, humiliation can also be understood as a sense of being emasculated—by the West, women, their fathers, culture, migrants, globalization, or peers. As has been shown, masculinity is a precarious status that must be continuously performed, reassured, and proved. Joining collective terrorism, as well as acting alone, offers perceived opportunities to re-establish and validate masculinity, however in exaggerated forms of destructive hypermasculinity.

To conclude, in addition to ideological, political, economic, regional, demographic, or psychological causes contributing to terrorism, experiences of threatened masculinity may be an underlying factor and driving force that contribute to better understanding of collective and lone actor terrorism.

Disclosures

Anne Maria Möller-Leimkühler does not have anything to disclose.

References

1. Schmidt, AP. The revised academic consensus definition of terrorism. *Perspectives on Terrorism*. 2012; **6**(2): 158–159.

2. Post, JM. Terrorism and right-wing extremism: the changing face of terrorism and political violence in the 21st century: the virtual community of hatred. *Int J Group Psychother*. 2015; **65**(2): 243–271.

3. Institute for Economics & Peace. Global terrorism index 2016. http://economicsand peace.org/wp-content/uploads/2016/11/Global-Terrorism-Index-2016.2.pdf?bcsi_sca n_64377d2312a1e457=0&bcsi_scan_filename=Global-Terrorism-Index-2016.2.pdf.

4. White, JR. *Terrorism and Homeland Security*, 7th ed. Belmont, CA: Wadsworth, Cengage Learning; 2012.

5. Bergen, P, Cruickshank, P. The Iraq effect: war has increased terrorism sevenfold worldwide. *Mother Jones*. 2007: 1–7. www.motherjones.com/politics/2007/03/iraq-effect-war-iraq-and-its-impact-war-terrorism-pg-2.

6. Pew Research Center. Unfavorable views of Jews and Muslims on the increase in Europe. www.pewglobal.org/2008/09/17/unfavorable-views-of-jews-and-muslims-on-the-increase-in-europe/. September 17, 2008.

7. Bremmer, I. These 5 facts explain why Europe is ground zero for terrorism. *Time*. http://time.com/4268579/brussels-attacks-islamist-terrorism-isis/. March 22, 2016.

8. Renard, T. Fear not: a critical perspective on the terrorist threat in Europe. Security Policy Brief No. 77; 2016. Egmont Royal Institute for International Relations, Brussels.

9. Niehoff, D. Not hardwired: the complex neurobiology of sex differences in violence. *Violence and Gender*. 2014; **1**(1): 19–24.

10. Staniloiu, A, Markowitsch, H. Gender differences in violence and aggression—a neurobiological perspective. *Procedia – Social and Behavioral Sciences*. 2012; **33**: 1032–1036.

11. Caspi, A, McClay, J, Miffitt, TE, et al. Role of genotype in the cycle of violence in maltreated children. *Science*. 2002; **297**(5582): 851–854.

12. Bogerts, B, Möller-Leimkühler, AM. Neurobiologische Ursachen und psychosoziale Bedingungen individueller Gewalt. *Nervenarzt*. 2013; **84**(11): 1329–1344.

13. Montoya, ER, Terburg, D, Bos, PA, van Honk, J. Testosterone, cortisol, and serotonin as key regulators of social aggression: a review and theoretical perspective. *Motiv Emot*. 2012; **36**(1): 65–73.

14. Walderhaug, E, Magnusson, A, Neumeister, A, et al. Interactive effects of sex and 5-HTTLPR on mood and impulsivity during tryptophan depletion in healthy people. *Biol Psychiatry*. 2007; **62**(6): 593–599.

15. Lighthall, NR, Mather, M, Gorlick, MA. Acute stress increases sex differences in risk seeking in the balloon analogue risk task. *PLoS ONE*. 2009; **4**(7): e6002.

16. Taylor, SE, Klein, LC, Lewis, BP, Gruenewald, TL, Gurung, RA, Updegraff, JA. Biobehavioral responses to stress in females: tend-and-befriend, not fight-or-flight. *Psychol Rev*. 2000; **107**(3): 411–429.

17. Stanton, SJ, Wirth, MM, Waugh, CE, Schultheiss, OC. Endogenous testosterone levels are associated with amygdala and ventromedial prefrontal cortex responses to anger faces in men but not women. *Biol Psychiatry*. 2009; **81**(2): 118–122.

18. Steinberg, L. A social neuroscience perspective on adolescent risk-taking. *Dev Rev*. 2008; **28**(1): 78–106.

19. Eaton, DK, Kann, L, Kinchen, S, et al. Youth risk behaviour surveillance – United States, 2011. *MMWR Surveill Summ*. 2012; **61**(4): 1–162.

20. Telzer, EH. Dopaminergic reward sensitivity can promote adolescent health: a new perspective on the mechanism of ventral striatum activation. *Dev Cogn Neurosci*. 2016; **17**: 57–67.

21. Goudie, C, Markoff, B. How ISIS recruiting videos mirror Hollywood scripts. http://abc7chicago.com/news/how-isis-recruiting-videos-mirror-hollywood-scripts/1194173/. February 9, 2016.

22. Riegler, T. Through the lenses of Hollywood: depictions of terrorism in American movies. *Perspectives on Terrorism*. 2010; **4**(2): 35–45.

23. Hall, A. ISIS has launched a new recruitment drive among unaccompanied youngsters in Germany's refugee camps. www.dailymail.co.uk/news/article-3799 915/ISIS-launched-new-recruitment-drive-unaccompanied-youngsters-Germany-s-refugee-camps-officials-warn-group-plots-Paris-style-carnage. September 21, 2016.

24. Connell, RW, Messerschmidt, JW. Hegemonic masculinity: rethinking the concept. *Gender and Society*. 2005; **19**(6): 829–859.

25. Holt, DB, Thompson, CJ. Man-of-action heroes: the pursuit of heroic masculinity in everyday consumption. *Journal of Consumer Research*. 2004; **31**(2): 425–440.

26. Ferber, AL, Kimmel, MS. The gendered face of terrorism. *Sociology Compass*. 2008; **2**(3): 870–887.

27. Bosson, JK, Vandello, JA. Precarious manhood and its links to action and aggression. *Current Directions in Psychological Science*. 2011; **20**(2): 82–86.

28. The Swedish Agency for Youth and Civil Society. Young and extreme—a youth and gender perspective on violent extremism. www.mucf.se/sites/default/files/publikationer_uploads/young-and-extreme.pdf. 2016.

29. Werner, F. Soldatische Männlichkeit im Vernichtungskrieg. Geschlechtsspezifische Dimensionen der Gewalt in Feldpostbriefen 1941–1944. In: Didczuneit V, Ebert J, Jander T, eds. *Schreiben im Krieg – Schreiben vom Krieg. Feldpost im Zeitalter der Weltkriege*. Essen, Germany: Klartext; 2011: 283–294.

30. Neizel, S, Welzer, H. *Soldaten: On Fighting, Killing and Dying: The Secret Second World War Tapes of German POWs*. New York, NY: Simon & Schuster/Paula Wiseman Books; 2012.

31. Morgan, DHJ. Theater of war: combat, the military, and masculinities. In: Brod H, Kaufman M, eds. *Theorizing Masculinities*. London: Sage; 1994: 165.

32. Eichler, M. Militarized masculinities in international relations. *Brown Journal of World Affairs*. 2014; **21**(1): 81–93.

33. McCue, C, Haahr, K. The impact of youth bulges on Islamist radicalization and violence. www.ctc.usma.edu/posts/the-impact-of-global-youth-bulges-on-islamist-radicalization-and-violence. 2008.

34. Cohen, D, Nusbett, RE, Bowdle, BF, Schwarz, N. Insult, aggression, and the southern culture of honor: an "experimental" ethnography. *J Pers Soc Psychol*. 1996; **70**(5): 945–959.

35. Richards, B. What drove Anders Breivik. *Contexts*. 2014; **13**(4): 42–47.

36. Junge, Männer. Die gefährlichste Spezies der Welt. Der Spiegel. 2008; 2. www.spiegel.de/spiegel/print/d-55294591.html.

37. Loeber, R, Hoeve, M, Slot, NW, van der Laan, PH. *Persisters and Desisters in Crime from Adolescence into Adulthood*. London: Routledge; 2012.

38. Newman, E. Exploring the "root causes" of terrorism. *Studies in Conflict & Terrorism*. 2006; **29**(8): 749–772.

39. Kivimäki, T, Montesanti, E. Global terrorism: causes, consequences and solutions. Global Research. www.globalresearch.ca/global-terrorism-causes-consequences-and-solutions/5529247. 2016.

40. Urdal, H. A clash of generations? Youth bulges and political violence. *International Studies Quarterly*. 2006; **50**(3): 607–629.

41. Aslam, M. *Gender-Based Explosions: The Nexus Between Muslim Masculinities, Jihadist Islamism and Terrorism*. Tokyo: United Nations University Press; 2012.

42. Gambetta, D, Hertog, S. *Engineers of Jihad: The Curious Connection Between Violent Extremism and Education*. Princeton, NJ: Princeton University Press; 2016.

43. Kivimäki, T. Executive summary. In: Kivimäki T, ed. *Development Cooperation as an Instrument in the Prevention of Terrorism*. Copenhagen: The Royal Danish Ministry of Foreign Affairs/Nordic Institute of Asia Studies; 2003.

44. Kroehnert, S, Klingholz, R. Not am Mann. Von Helden der Arbeit zur neuen Unterschicht? Berlin Institut für Bevölkerung und Entwicklung .www.berlin-institut .org/fileadmin/user_upload/Studien/Not_am_Mann_Webversion.pdf. 2007.

45. Kroehnert, S, Vollmer, S. Where have all young women gone? Gender-specific migration from East to West Germany. World Development Report. Background Paper. http://siteresources.worldbank.org/INTWDR2009/Resources/4231006–1204741572978/Vollmer.pdf. 2008.

46. Koehler, D. Right-wing extremism and terrorism in Europe. *PRISM*. 2016; **6**(2): 85–104.

47. Sageman, M. Understanding terror networks. Foreign Policy Research Institute. www.fpri.org/enotes/20041101.middleeast.sageman.understandingterrornetworks.html. 2004.

48. McGilloway, A, Ghosh, P, Bhui, K. A systematic review of pathways to and processes associated with radicalization and extremism amongst Muslims in Western societies. *Int Rev Psychiatry*. 2015; **27**(1): 39–50.

49. Möller-Leimkühler, AM, Bogerts, B. Kollektive Gewalt. Neurobiologische, psychosoziale und gesellschaftliche Bedingungen. *Nervenarzt*. 2013; **84**(11): 1345–1358.

50. Tajfel, H, Turner, J. An integrative theory of intergroup conflict. In: Hogg MA, Abrams D, eds. *Intergroup Relations*. New York, NY: Psychology Press; 2001: 94–109.

51. Tajfel, H. Experiments in intergroup discrimination. *Scientific American*. 1970; **223**: 96–102.

52. Swann, WB, Jetten, J, Gómez, A, Whitehouse, H. When group membership gets personal: a theory of identity fusion. *Psychol. Rev*. 2012; **119**(3): 441–456.

53. Swann, WB, Buhrmester, MD. Identity fusion. *Current Directions in Psychological Science*. 2015; **24**(1): 52–57.

54. Atran, S, Henrich, J. The evolution of religion: how cognitive by-products, adaptive learning heuristics, ritual displays, and group competition generate deep commitments to prosocial religions. *Biological Theory*. 2010; **5**(1): 18–30.

55. Atran, S. The devoted actor: unconditional commitment and intractable conflict across cultures. *Current Anthropology*. 2016; **57**(13): S192–S203.

56. Abrahms, M. What terrorists really want. *International Security*. 2008; **32**(4): 78–105.

57. Marneros, A. *Hitlers Urenkel. Rechtsradikale Gewalttäter*. Bern, Switzerland: Scherz; 2002.

58. Simi, P, Windisch, S, Sporer, K. *Recruitment and Radicalization Among US Far Right Terrorists*. College Park, MD: START; 2016.

59. Sitzer, P, Heitmeyer, W. Right-wing extremist violence among adolescents in Germany. *New Dir Youth Dev*. 2008; **2008**(119): 169–185.

60. Pantucci, R, Ellis, C, Chaplais, L. *Lone-Actor Terrorism: Literature Review*. The Royal United Services Institute for Defense and Security Studies. London, UK: Stephen Austin and Sons; 2015.

61. Weimann, G. Lone wolves in cyberspace. *Journal of Terrorism Research*. 2012; **3**(2): 75–90.

62. Gill, P, Horgan, J, Deckert, P. Bombing alone: tracing the motivations and antecedent behaviors of lone-actor terrorists. *J Forensic Sci*. 2014; **59**(2): 425–435.

63. McCauley, C, Moskalenko, S, Van Son, B. Characteristics of lone-wolf violent offenders: a comparison of assassins and school attackers. *Perspectives on Terrorism*. 2013; **7**(1): 4–24.

64. Hamm, M, Spaaj, R. Lone wolf terrorism in America: using knowledge of radicalization pathways to forge prevention strategies. Final Report. www.ncjrs.gov/pdffiles1/nij/grants/248691. 2015.

65. Gill, P. *Lone-Actor Terrorists: A Behavioural Analysis*. London: Routledge; 2015.

66. Borum, R. Informing lone-offender investigations. *Criminology & Public Policy*. 2013; **12**(1): 103–112.

67. Corner, E, Gill, P. A false dichotomy? Mental illness and lone-actor terrorism. *Law Hum Behav*. 2015; **39**(1): 23–34.

68. Gruenewald, J, Chermak, S, Freilich, JD. Distinguishing "loner" attacks from other domestic extremist violence. *Criminology & Public Policy*. 2013; **12**(1): 65–91.

69. Langman, P. *Amok im Kopf. Warum Schüler töten*. Weinheim, Germany: Beltz; 2009.

70. Böckler, N, Hoffmann, J, Zick, A. The Frankfurt Airport attack: a case study on the radicalization of a lone-actor terrorist. *Journal of Threat Assessment and Management*. 2015; **2**(3–4): 153–163.

71. Theweleit, K. *Das Lachen der Täter*. Breivik u.a. St. Pölten–Salzburg–Wien: Residenz Verlag; 2. Auflage; 2015.

72. SPIEGEL. Can Europe's populists be blamed for Anders Breivik's crusade? www .spiegel.de/international/europe/the-trail-of-evil-can-europe-s-populists-be-blamed-for-anders-breivik-s-crusade-a-777710.html. August 1, 2011.

73. Forsythe, P. Profiling ideology the best way to combat terrorism. http://thebattleoftours .blogspot.de/2016/04/profiling-ideology-best-way-to-combat.html. April 11, 2016.

74. Goldhagen, DJ. The humiliation myth. *Democracy Journal*. http://democracyjour nal.org/magazine/4/the-humiliation-myth/. 2007.

Religion, Violence, and the Brain: a Neuroethical Perspective

Alberto Carrara

Introduction

I think it's educationally pernicious to fill children's minds up with falsehoods when the truth is so exciting, about the nature of the universe, where it comes from, things like that. We're so close to understanding it. But also, of course, religions—not all of them, but some of them—inspire people to do terrible deeds. Because of faith, which by definition requires no evidence. It can be used to justify suicide bombings, beheading apostates, stoning people to death.[1]

This quote comes from a personal communication of Richard Dawkins to Raphael Lataster. It is easy to perceive from Dawkins' statement a Western widespread stereotype that links religions with evil, antisocial behaviors. It is not so unusual to hear that religions lead to division, hatred, war, and other evil behaviors in society. The background of this way of thinking on religion and on religious people is at least twofold. From one side, it emphasizes a diachronic portrait of history and philosophy of religion in which this human factor is considered always present when great wars took place, or when atrocities, such as genocides, massacres of ethnics groups, etc., were carried out. This sort of causal correlation, evil happens–people who commit the crime are religious, is very common and is due to the fact that at least 84 per cent of the world's population belongs to a religion.[2]

From another perspective, the same stereotype that correlates religion with evil behaviors is based on a false premise that struggles to impose a radical and constitutive dichotomy between science and faith: the so-called "opposition paradigm."[3] According to this belief, only empirical science can achieve and teach "truth," the only and absolute truth based on evidence; instead, the central pillar of religion, faith, requiring no scientific evidence, would fill people's minds up with falsehoods.

The controversies over religion being the cause of terrorism and evil behaviors are serious, and extensive effort is required to separate the wheat from the chaff.

Therefore, the first term that we need to clarify is "religion." For sure, it is a crucial inquiry what a religion is, particularly to Religious Studies scholars. Following Hubert Seiwert, we recognize that for most of the twentieth century, theory in the study of religion was marked by two main approaches: (1) theologically or philosophically informed phenomenology, and (2) social-scientific theories of religion. It was only in the last decade of the twentieth century that a third school of interpretation became prevalent: (3) theories inspired by the natural sciences, predominantly evolutionary biology, cognitive psychology, psychoanalysis, and nowadays neuroscience.[4] Along these lines of speculation, Loyal Rue attempts to combine all three of these approaches and, at the end, he sees religion as a natural phenomenon that is a by-product of the evolution of the human brain, a sort of a product of biological and cultural evolution with the utmost adaptive value for survival and the well-being of the human species. Starting from almost the same premises as Richard Dawkins' biological interpretation of religions, Rue's theory considers religion not as the major obstacle to human flourishing, but instead, as a crucial factor in mankind's development and a concrete means of enhancing the universal human nature that can be known by examining the evolutionary history of humankind.[5,6,7]

A Neuro-anthropological Framework

Taking these considerations in mind, let us move towards some anthropological distinctions in the context of neuroethics.

According to Levy and Clausen's colossal Springer Handbook (2015), neuroethics "is systematic and informed reflection on and interpretation of neuroscience, and related sciences of the mind (psychology in all its many forms, psychiatry, artificial intelligence, and so on), in order to understand its implications for human self-understanding and perils and prospects of its applications."[8] An interesting field of neuroethical reflexion deals with what is known as "neuroscience of religion" or "neurotheology" or "spiritual neuroscience" which studies the relationship between religious experiences and brain functions[9–11] in order to go deep in understanding this central query: is our brain hardwired to produce God, or is our brain hardwired to perceive God?[12] In our concrete topic, neuroethical interdisciplinary reflection can help to explain a little bit more the plausible genesis of evil and terrorism behaviors, contextualizing them in our complex multidimensional constitution. The challenging question of how to explain evil behaviors remains unresolved. Far from a merely mono-factorial reductionist model of explanation of human reality, present and future research is calling to move from a one-to-one causal explanation to a complex and interdependent multifactors system analysis. This wager needs not only interdisciplinarity, which implies the interaction of different disciplines coming from the same methodological framework, but also multidisciplinarity, which points towards a real dialogue and integration between different types of rationality: from an empirical one to the realm of sociology, economy, law, philosophy, and even theology.

In contemporary neuroethical thought, the human being, the individual, is considered to be a psychosomatic entity,[12] a minded-animal[13] (Aristotle defined man as a rational animal, while contemporary philosophical anthropology sees us as "incarnate-spirit"[14]). We are an intrinsic and extrinsically inter-relational organism, in which our mental activities are dynamically embodied and embedded in the frame of our living system behaving in our concrete environmental culture.[15] This ecological view of the human mind and body (brain) as both being embodied and embedded in the relation of the living organism and its cultural milieu takes the technical denomination of the bio(neuro)-psycho-social-spiritual model.[16,17] The human consists of multiple levels and dimensions of existence: from physical and biological to psychological and spiritual ones.[12] The human body, and the brain as its fundamental part, is a biological, open system that maintains itself (homeostasis) in a constantly changing environment. From the time it was structured during embryogenesis to the moment of physical death, the brain is involved in a continuous formation and reshaping through a plethora of factors. This mediating organ of human experience, action and interaction, integrating the macroscopic dimension of the living organism and its interactions and experiences with the microscopic facet of bio-physical reactions, may also be considered as "a matrix that transforms all experience into lasting dispositions of behaviour and experience," as psychiatrist Thomas Fuchs constantly pointed out in his reflections.[10]

This ecological and dynamic anthropological perspective, neuroscientifically based, has the advantage of avoiding the two main stands—at least—that are responsible for de-humanizing medical care: (1) the dualistic nature of the biomedical model, with its drastic separation of body and mind considered in a Cartesian substantive way; (2) the excessively materialistic and reductionist orientation of medical thinking leading to an exclusive consideration of human being as a pure machine (along with 1747 Julien Offray de la Mettrie's *L'homme machine* or contemporary 1983 Jean-Pierre Changeux's *L'homme neuronal*).[11]

In this neuroethical context, consciousness/mind/spirit, from one side, and brain/body/matter, from the other, are conceived in a unity-dual way (not dualism) as "different sides of the same phenomenon, neither reducible to each other."[12] According to an anti-reductionist approach, this model allows integration of "the emergence of a form of causation distinctive from physics where mental/conscious agency (a) is neither identical with nor reducible to brain processes and (b) does exert 'downward' causal influence on brain plasticity and the various levels of brain functioning."[12]

Separating The Wheat from The Chaff: Some Distinctions in The Context of Religion

Taking into account this framework, we may consider the human being's development in an unceasing tension between three poles: (1) the dimension of being (nature), (2) the mental facet of thinking and feeling, and (3) the bodily side of behaving.

The human species *Homo sapiens* is also defined as a religious animal (*Homo religiosus*), as anthropologist Julien Ries pointed out.[18] The first distinction takes place at the level of being, in this case, being religious or "religiosity": through history humanity manifests and expresses this nature by means of ideas (religious beliefs), feelings (religious emotions), and religious behaviors, such as cave paintings, images, symbols, and rituals (dimension of behaving or acting).

Religions are specific and concrete forms of organization of all these human dimensions. They can be defined as paths that have the potential of improving good thoughts, feelings, and behaviors, fostering human flourishing, as well as a harmonic development of societies.

"Good and Evil" Hardwired Brains

A recent meta-analysis focusing on prosociality across 93 studies and 11,653 participants recognized some significant aspects of religions: (1) the fact that religious beliefs and behaviors are ubiquitous features of human lives; (2) religious reminders have prosocial effects (religious prosociality); (3) religion is actually one concrete path to prosociality, not an exclusive one, but yes a cofactor that has the potential to contribute to the positive effect of enhancing prosocial and emphatic behaviors: religion may cause people to act more prosocially; (4) of course, as a human aspect, prosociality tends to have multifactorial causes; (5) a prosocial disposition may cause people to become religious; (6) variables, such as compassion or guilt, may increase both religiosity and prosociality; and (7) the evidence that aspects of religious beliefs and rituals motivate people to sacrifice self-interest for others.[19] The authors of this study pointed out a significant statement: "We found clear support for religious priming in samples drawn from populations culturally shaped by the highly influential prosocial religious traditions of the Abrahamic faiths, comprising a majority of the world's population, where we would expect religious concepts to influence prosociality."[13]

Although the origin of religious prosociality still needs more comprehensive and interdisciplinary studies, the distinctions just outlined, taken together with a growing clinical neuroscientific literature dealing with neurobiology and neurophysiology of evil behaviors[20] and neural correlates of religious beliefs and experiences,[12,21] may contribute to structure an integrative picture in order to clarify better the role of religion in the genesis of human evil behaviors ("evil hardwired brains"), such as terrorist attacks and suicide bombers, and to propose some ethical means to foster "good hardwired brains" in a globalized society which are going to enhance human flourishing, harmony, peace, and being.

A neurobiological perspective on evil behaviors may take into consideration this threefold brain dynamic: (1) loss of connectivity or dissociation of cortico-striatal processing from limbic input, which is one of the main neurophysiological underpinnings of a psychopath's traits (extremely rational but poorly empathetic); (2) hyperactivation of limbic processing, resulting in hyper-instinctive responses; and (3) cortical orbitofrontal reduction, which fosters a deprivation of normal rational control over primitive instincts and passions.[22–25]

Here is a brief summary of a plausible dynamic development of what we may call a "good brain" and an "evil brain." Usually "good" and "evil" are terms that specify a quality of some human actions according to a shared ethical system of norms. Here we understand them as different types of brain configurations (morphology and functionality) that in accordance with several other factors predispose an individual to behave in a certain way.

Together with other positive co-enhancers, such as a good gestation period, a positive childhood, an enriched cultural and social environment where justice and cooperation among others are considered values to live and to promote, etc., a "good brain" (a proper developed and healthy nervous system) is a key element of human flourishing that, at the end, contributes to produce prosocial behaviors.

An "evil brain," instead, is the opposite configuration, a sort of necessary prerequisite, that together with other pharmacological, cultural, and social co-factors structures an "evil psychology" that may end up causing evil behaviors.

A Plausible Dynamic

At the origin, moving from the religious nature of human being (being religious or "religiosity") through a process of biological development, the organism structures a nervous system that is able to sustain higher mental and affective functions, such as religious thinking (beliefs), religious feelings and emotions. Inside a specific cultural and social environment, these higher human activities are shaped by a specific and concrete form of organization of religious beliefs and rituals, namely a religion. This complexity, through the phenomenon of plasticity, and in cooperation with a lot of other positive factors, contributes to wire a "good brain" that allows the individual to behave in a prosocial fashion, while fostering good values for the sake and good of his/her flourishing, and the harmony, peace, and well-being of the whole society.

There is a growing scientific literature pointing towards clinical benefits of religious practices, such as prayers, meditation, introspection, forms of relaxation and breathing, postures and gestures, and so on, especially in end-of-life and palliative care.[26] Religiosity is considered a key factor involved in the management of health and diseases and patient longevity.[27] A funny single case study using functional MRI has recently involved as a participant a Catholic German bishop of 72 years. This research suggested that a highly religious person trained in contemplation rewired his brain in such a way to constantly behave in a peaceful, calm, and relaxed fashion.[28] A lot of brain areas and psychological functions associated with them were studied during religious experiences.[12] Neuroscientific evidence supports that religions and religious practices play a key role in shaping a "good brain" structure. Therefore, religions and religious practices have the potential to provide benefits to our brain and by shaping it they could have a positive impact on health and well-being. For those reasons, the spiritual dimension of human being (religiosity) became part of the bio-psycho-social model for the care of patients at the end of life.[29]

Now let's consider another situation. When the same developmental dynamic takes place, but a manipulation of a religious trait—or many—perpetrated by an "evil leader"[30]—or many—(a dictator, for instance, who uses religion for the sake of conquering and preserving power), is promoted, the results may be very different. Together with other factors of vulnerability, such as psychopharmacological drug abuse, violence, child abuse, social and economic degradation, psychopathic traits, fundamentalism, and so on, those manipulations of religious aspects might shape and wire a vulnerable nervous system towards an "evil brain" configuration that unfortunately may result in violent behaviors, murders, atrocities, and suicidal terroristic attacks. Manipulations of some religious traits by "evil leaders" within a concrete religious framework or a specific culture shaped by a religion may have a twofold consequence: (1) an attractor effect, that is, "natural" recruitment of psycho-vulnerable people; (2) negatively rewiring vulnerable nervous systems, which together with other socioeconomic factors (not excluding pharmacological abuse) contribute in shaping "evil brains."

The authors of the recent meta-analysis focusing on prosociality mentioned previously also emphasized the fact that religious concepts taken in the wrong way may have the power to encourage uncharitable attitudes, such as racism; therefore, they established a line of dependence of culturally transmitted religious beliefs on cognitive activation.[17] One of the most powerful religious concepts or religious beliefs is, for sure, the complex idea of God or the so-called "image of God." At this level, there is the risk for every religion to lead towards an absolutistic and fundamentalist conception of the divinity. By influencing a concrete way of thinking about God or divinity, groups of evil subjects, such as nowadays' Isis leaders, foster this kind of brain deconstruction, especially in vulnerable people such as children and adolescents.

The plausible model just summarized can help us to understand that one key factor that may contribute to the evil that springs along history from religious people is not religions themselves, nor religiosity, but evil manipulations of the "image of God."

Linking religion with terrorism because conceivable radicalizations of religious traits actually foster terroristic attacks sounds like saying that science is accountable for atomic bomb devastations, or that politics is responsible for dictatorial systems.

A Final Remark

Religions have to be considered to be personal and public enhancers, instead of enemies. Society and institutions have a duty to foster and integrate in lay educational training programs all good religious values, attitudes, and behaviors, in place of eliminating them. In a cosmopolitan context, it is not easy to see how we can democratically eliminate the undoubted value of religions in the flourishing of individuals who freely chose to believe in a concrete faith.

In a recently developing field of neuroethics called moral enhancement, authors, such as Persson and Savulescu, idealized interventions consisting in genetic modifications, neural implants, or pharmaceuticals, with the intention to re-setting both "normal" and "evil brains" in order to promote morally good behaviors and prevent humanity from devastation due to climate change and terrorism.[31] Despite much skepticism derived from analyzing such proposals using an agential risk agenda,[32] there are other, more realistic neuroethical perspectives engaging and harnessing neuroscientific and neurotechnological (the so-called "neuroS/T") development with at least a twofold purpose: (1) to achieve the "3 Ps' hope": to predict, to prevent, and to protect against acts of terrorism, serial killings, mass massacres, genocides, and so on; and (2) "to guide right and sound applications of neuroS/T to 'deliver us from evil' while not being led into temptations of ampliative claims and inapt use."[33] Proposals dealing with the employment of neuroS/T to fulfill those expectations, both attractive and tempting, are of course profoundly constrained by technical, practical, and neuroethical limitations. Giordano et al. established clear neuroethical postulates that we need to integrate in our reflection on "religion, violence, and brains" in order to avoid easy and comfortable reductionism about the religious dimension of mankind. Such pillars are: "(1) aggressiveness is not an explicitly diagnostic term or status; (2) aggressiveness does not necessarily evoke or culminate in frank inter-personal and/or social violence; (3) even a condition characterized by aggression, anti-social, and inter-personal violence—such as psychopathy—does not uniformly present such traits; (4) predisposition does not infer expression; and (5) perhaps most importantly, correlation does not infer causality."[27]

In the future, neuroS/T may help us to detect vulnerable subjects who are going to develop "evil brain" configurations, preventing them from performing evil behaviors, and in the end, protecting citizens. Such types of neuro-applications may also become coercion tools, instead of a means for social ransom or redemption, in particular, because they could be received passively, without motivation by vulnerable people.

The key discrimination factor here is the personal and integrative engagement in order to stably rewire a vulnerable brain.

NeuroS/T alone are going to miss the target. They need to be included in the multidimensional anthropological model depicted above. The latter puts forward an integral view where the human being is seen as a uni-duality organism, a psychosomatic entity consisting of multiple levels of existence: physical, biological, psychological, and spiritual.[12]

This contemporary neuroethical attempt may provide new insights in order to: (1) draw distinctions between different dimensions inside "religions"; (2) highlight plausible neuro and psycho-religious enhancement effects; and (3) distinguish them from evil manipulations and exploitations.

A multi-religious globalized society that wants to "deliver us from evil" needs to combine and include all human dimensions, including good religious values and behaviors. As a final example, "Religions for Peace" is the world's largest and most representative multi-religious coalition that advances common action among the world's religious communities to transform violent conflict, advance human development, promote just and harmonious societies, and protect the earth.

Religions, with their spiritual and moral resources, may play a concrete role and responsibility in building peace and justice, promoting fraternity, disarmament and care for ecology, and in eradication of terrorism and violence.

Disclosures

The author does not have any disclosures, and the author does not have any affiliation with or financial interest in any organization that might pose a conflict of interest

References

1. Lataster, R. A superscientific definition of 'religion' and a clarification of Richard Dawkins' New Atheism. *Literature & Aesthetics*. 2014; **24**(2): 109–124.

2. According to the Pew Research Center, the statistics in 2015 is the following: 84 per cent religious (subdivided as such: 31.2 per cent Christians; 24.1 per cent Muslims; 15.1 per cent Hindus; 6.9 per cent Buddhists; 5.7 per cent Folk religions; 0.8 per cent others; 0.2 per cent Jews) and 16 per cent classified as "unaffiliated." www.pew research.org/fact-tank/2017/04/05/christians-remain-worlds-largest-religious -group-but-they-are-declining-in-europe/.

3. Park, JZ. Conflict between religion and science among academic scientists? *J Sci Study Religion.* 2009; **48**(2): 276–292.

4. Seiwert, H. Theory of religion as myth. On Loyal Rue (2005), Religion is not about God. In: Stausberg M, ed. *Contemporary Theories of Religion. A Critical Companion.* New York, NY: Routledge; 2009: 224–241.

5. Rue, L. *Religion Is Not About God: How Spiritual Traditions Nurture Our Biological Nature and What To Expect When They Fail.* New Brunswick: Rutgers University Press; 2005.

6. Rue, L. Religious naturalism – where does it lead? *Zygoll.* 2007; **42**(2): 409–422.

7. Schilbrack K. *Philosophy and the Study of Religions: A Manifesto.* Malden, MA: Wiley-Blackwell; 2014: 128.

8. Clausen, J, Levy, N, eds. *Handbook of Neuroethics.* New York, NY: Springer; 2015.

9. Whitfield, W. Towards a neurotheology? *Int J Psychiatr Nurs Res.* 2003; **8**(3): 941.

10. Shukla, S, Acharya, S, Rajput, D. Neurotheology – matters of the mind or matters that mind? *J Clin Diagn Res JCDR.* 2013; 7(7): 1486–1490.

11. Sayadmansour, A. Neurotheology: the relationship between brain and religion. *Iran J Neurol.* 2014; **13**(1): 52–55.

12. Fingelkurts, AA, Fingelkurts AA. Is our brain hardwired to produce God, or is our brain hardwired to perceive God? A systematic review on the role of the brain in mediating religious experience. *Cogn Process.* 2009; **10**(4): 293–326.

13. Gabriel, M. *I am Not a Brain. Philosophy of Mind for the Twenty-First Century.* Cambridge: Polity Press; 2017.

14. Lucas, R. *Man Incarnate Spirit. A Philosophy of Man Compendium.* Turin: Circle Press; 2008.

15. Fuchs, T. The brain – a mediating organ. *J Consc Studies.* 2011; **18**(7–8): 196–221.

16. Borrell-Carrió, F, Suchman AL, Epstein RM. The biopsychosocial model 25 years later: principles, practice, and scientific inquiry. *Ann Family Med.* 2004; **2**(6): 576–582.

17. Beerbower, E, Winters, D, Kondrat, D. Bio-psycho-social-spiritual needs of adolescents and young adults with life-threatening illnesses: implications for social work practice. *Soc Work Health Care.* 2018; **29**: 1–17.

18. Ries, J. *The Origins of Religions.* Grand Rapids, MI: Eerdmans Pub Co.; 1994.

19. Shariff, AF, Willard, AK, Andersen, T, Norenzayan, A. Religious priming: a meta-analysis with a focus on prosociality. *Pers Soc Psychol Rev.* 2016; **20**(1): 27–48.

20. Stein, DJ. The neurobiology of evil: psychiatric perspectives on perpetrators. *Ethn Health.* 2000; **5**(3–4): 303–315.

21. Harris, S, Kaplan, JT, Curiel, A, et al. The neural correlates of religious and non-religious belief. *PLoS ONE.* 2009; **4**(10): 1–9.

22. Yang, Y, Narr, KL, Baker, LA, et al. Frontal and striatal alterations associated with psychopathic traits in adolescents. *Psychiatry Res.* 2015; **231**(3): 333–340.

23. Pape, LE, Cohn, MD, Caan, MW, et al. Psychopathic traits in adolescents are associated with higher structural connectivity. *Psychiatry Res.* 2015; **233**(3): 474–480.

24. Yang, Y, Wang, P, Baker, LA, et al. Thicker temporal cortex associates with a developmental trajectory for psychopathic traits in adolescents. *PLOS ONE.* 2015; **10**(5): 1–15.

25. Rogers, JC, De Brito, SA. Cortical and subcortical gray matter volume in youths with conduct problems: a meta-analysis. *JAMA Psychiatry.* 2016; **73**(1): 64–72.

26. Agarwal, S, Kumar, V, Agarwal, S, et al. Meditational spiritual intercession and recovery from disease in palliative care: a literature review. *Ann Palliat Med.* 2018; **7**(1): 41–62.

27. Mishra, SK, Togneri, E, Tripathi, B, Trikamji, B. Spirituality and religiosity and its role in health and diseases. *J Relig Health.* 2017; **56**(4): 1282–1301.

28. Silveira, S, Bao, Y, Wang, L, et al. Does a bishop pray when he prays? And does his brain distinguish between different religions? *PsyCh J.* 2015; **4**: 199–207.

29. Sulmasy, DP. A biopsychosocial-spiritual model for the care of patients at the end of life. *Gerontologist.* 2002; **42**(3): 24–33.

30. Marazziti, D. Psychiatry and terrorism: exploring the unacceptable. *CNS Spectrums.* 2016; **21**: 128–130.

31. Persson, I, Savulescu, J. *Unfit for the Future: The Need for Moral Enhancement.* Oxford: Oxford University Press; 2012.

32. Torres, P. Moral bioenhancement and agential risks: good and bad outcomes. *Bioethics.* 2017; **31**(9): 691–696.

33. Giordano, J, Kulkarni, A, Farwell, J. Deliver us from evil? The temptation, realities, and neuroethico-legal issues of employing assessment neurotechnologies in public safety initiatives. *Theor Med Bioeth.* 2014; **35**(1): 73–89.

Chapter

8

Brain Alterations Potentially Associated with Aggression and Terrorism

Bernhard Bogerts, Maria Schöne, and
Stephanie Breitschuh

Introduction

Between 1971 and 1993, Germany's most notorious terrorist group, the Red Army Faction (RAF), killed 33 people and injured more than 200 others, among them many representatives of the justice system, the political establishment, and the economy. The intellectual head of this left lunatic fringe group was Ulrike Meinhof. Before she entered the RAF in 1970, she was a well-known and recognized journalist who committed herself by peaceful means to promote her political ideas. Before she joined the RAF, she underwent neurosurgery in 1962 after developing neurological symptoms because of a vascular tumor (angioma) at the base of her brain next to the right medial temporal lobe. In the years after this surgery, she developed a change of personality that included increasingly aggressive traits. She later wrote the "The Concept of the Urban Guerilla," by which she tried to adapt the strategies of South American guerilla groups to West German cities. After she was captured, she committed suicide in 1976 during the court proceedings against leading members of the RAF. An autopsy of her brain was performed, and the neuropathologist described small circumscribed damage to the cortical tissue and adjoining white matter in the right anterior medial temporal lobe, very close to the amygdala, as a result of the brain surgery she had in 1962, but no damage to other brain structures.[1] Her brain lesion was localized in a key limbic region involved in neuronal control of basic emotions, including aggressive and violent behaviors. The content of the radical political ideas she fought for can of course not be explained by the postsurgical limbic brain damage but are rather a result of the special political and social environment of her time. However, the fact that she developed a personality change with increasing aggressiveness and violence has to be regarded as a result of the brain injury closely related to the amygdala. This regionally localized type of brain damage might not be representative for terroristic behavior in general, but we are not aware of any other postmortem or neuroimaging investigation of a terrorist's brain.

To our knowledge, with two exceptions, there are also no autopsy findings in persons who ran amok. The best-documented historic case of an amok runner, at least in European psychiatry, belongs to the teacher Ernst Wagner, who in 1913 first killed his wife and 4 children, then burned down several buildings, and then shot and killed 9 male inhabitants and injured 11 others during one night in a village near the city of Stuttgart. Months before the mass killings, he began to train himself to shoot pistols. He was eventually over-powered and subdued during the course of his mass murder spree and then examined by a psychiatrist, who diagnosed him as suffering from paranoia, since for years he had felt persecuted and threatened by his victims. After he died years later in a forensic hospital, a brain autopsy revealed a small circumscribed lesion in the left anterior entorhinal cortex, next to the hippo-campus and amygdala, while other parts of the brain looked inconspicuous.[1]

The second case of a person who ran amok and underwent a brain autopsy was Charles Whitman, a 25-year-old college student at the University of Texas. In 1966, he first stabbed his mother and his wife, and he then shot and killed 17 people from his sniper's nest in the university tower, injuring 32 others. Months before the shootings, he sought psychiatric help because he was suffering from increasing personal stress and psychological isolation. He felt that something was going wrong in his head, and in his suicide note he requested that an autopsy be performed to determine if something had changed in his brain. After he was shot by security forces at the top of the tower, an autopsy was indeed performed. Aside from many of his brain parts being damaged by penetrating fragments of bone created by his gunshot wounds, a small tumor (a glioblastoma) was found beneath the thalamus, impinging upon the hypothalamus and compressing the amygdala.[2,3]

Neuronal Correlates of Violence

The brain lesions in these three well-known cases have at least one thing in common: they were located in limbic structures of the anterior temporal lobe involved in the neuronal control of amygdala activities and, via the amygdala, also of the hypothalamic and lower brainstem areas, called by MacLean the "reptilian brain."[4] In these phylogenetically very old brain structures, groups of neurons are located that play a central role in the brain networks respon-sible for aggressive behavior and thus can be regarded as some kind of neuronal "generators" of aggression. Already in 1932, the Swiss physiologist Hess could demonstrate in cats that electrical stimulation of hypothalamic and other regions of the "reptilian brain" immediately provoked aggressive behavior.[5,6] Years later, these experiments were extended by Ploog,[7] who detected cell groups in the medial hypothalamus and medial amygdala related to the *reactive/defensive rage type* of aggression. The *proactive/predatory attack type* of aggression was elicited by stimulation of cell groups in the lateral hypothalamus and lateral amygdala. Under certain physiological conditions, these cell groups in the medial and lateral hypothalamus come into action if either threatening environmental conditions or aggression-inducing cue stimuli activate them via fiber tracts from the amygdala. Under pathological conditions, certain brain diseases can cause abnormal activation or a lack of inhibition of these cell groups by afferent fibers from the limbic or cortical association areas[8] or, as shown in the experiments of Hess and Ploog, if they are activated experimentally by direct electrical stimulation. Even in humans, electrical stimulation of the amygdala, performed for diagnostic purposes before stereotactic surgery in patients suffering from temporal lobe epilepsy, has caused severe impulsive aggressive outbursts.[9] Already in 1937, Klüver and Bucy[10] showed that their quite aggressive monkeys after destruction of the anterior temporal lobe (including the amygdala) displayed a "psychic blindness" characterized by a lack of anxiety and by steadily tame behavior.

Aside from temporal lobe epilepsy, which is caused by abnormal neuronal discharges in temporolimbic groups of neurons and is sometimes associated with sudden violent acts, limbic structures in the medial temporal lobe also belong to the regions that exhibit more or less subtle structural or functional damage in a significant proportion of patients suffering from psychotic diseases (e.g., schizophrenia),[11,12] which might explain the increased frequency of aggressive attacks in such psychotic syndromes.[13]

The neuronal generators of violence in the limbic system and hypothalamus did not arise incidentally: they are—aside from neuronal networks for prosocial attitudes—a product of a long evolutionary process that provided for the more aggressive male individuals or species an advantage in reproducing themselves while diminishing this chance for their victims. It has been shown that the primates (including *Homo sapiens*), among all the vertebrata, have the highest rates of killing members of their own species, with about 2 per cent dying as the result of an attack from their own group or from other human groups.[14] Moreover, hostile and martial attitudes against other groups combined with parochial altruistic behavior for in-group members also provide a strong evolutionary advantage.[15] Thus, neuronal substrates that are responsible for violence belong to the phylogenetically old equipment present in the brains of the human species in general.

Do Terrorists Have a Peculiar Neurobiological Predisposition?

There are several reasons to assume that at least a significant proportion of terrorist brains has a biological predisposition to violent behavior, so that one can conclude that the various ideologies claimed by them as justification for their terrorist acts are not the real reason for their behavior. Such adverse early life experiences as misuse in childhood, oppressive education, and lack of positive parental emotional attention, which are frequently characteristic of violent offenders, have plastic effects on such limbic brain regions as the amygdala and hippocampus. They cause not only enduring psychological scars but also long-lasting functional and even structural changes in the brain.[16] A large body of evidence also demonstrates the considerable influence of genes for the emergence of aggressive personality traits, psychopathy, and even religious fundamentalism.[17] Adoption studies and investigations of identical twins have shown that genetic factors may explain up to 50 per cent of the causative variance of criminal offences.[18,19] Among the genetic components showing an affinity for aggressive behavior, the monoamine oxidase A (MAOA) gene received special attention.[20,21] The low-expression variant of this gene has a particularly high affinity for violent behavior, especially if it occurs in combination with traumatic childhood experiences.[22] Moreover, abnormalities in neurotransmitters, especially serotonin, and hormones (testosterone, cortisol, vasopressin) seem to contribute to the etiology of aggressive traits (for a review, see Rosell and Siever[23]).

On the other hand, there are many historical examples (see, e.g., Browning[24]) that previously completely ordinary men without any signs of abnormal psychology have committed war crimes, atrocities, and genocide due to a mixture of motives, including the group dynamics of conformity, deference to authority, role adaptation, and alteration of moral norms. It has also been shown that randomly selected normal people under special conditions of psychological experiments are able to willingly perform cruelties if they are told to do so by authorities or if they are allowed to do so as custodians.[25–28] This shows that without a neurobiological predisposition or brain pathology, particular psychosocial constellations and/or group dynamics can give rise to violent acts. This is especially the case for various forms of individual and collective aggression.[29]

Individuals who join terror groups very often have a history of a previous criminal career. Analyzing the case histories of 784 persons in Germany who joined the so-called Islamic State of Iraq and the Levant (ISIL) between 2012 and 2015, it was found that two-thirds of these overwhelmingly male persons were known to the police because of violence, property offences, or political criminal acts.[30] In fact, more than half had committed three or more criminal offences before joining ISIL. It was reasoned that, because of their inherent readiness to violence, such persons search for suitable ideologies under which to act out their tendencies to harm, injure, and kill. From a neurobiological point of view, it seems justified to assume that the neuronal generators of aggression and violence in the human "reptilian brain" and limbic system are either per se more active in such persons by genetic or biographical influences or that they are less inhibited by brain systems that are normally responsible for such prosocial attitudes as empathy and compassion. The latter could again be the consequence of predisposing genes, but also of various pathological brain abnormalities (among them, brain tissue defects by injury, atrophy, viral infection, tumors or innate hypoplasias, or psychoses); antisocial, fanatic, and/or paranoid personality disorders; or of a character trait called "psychopathy," that is, a callous antisocial lifestyle with no intellectual defects but displaying a typical inability to have a sense of the value of others. There are reports that about 40 per cent of the lone wolves (lone-acting terrorists) who develop their hateful ideologies without contact with any particular terrorist group are suffering from a psychiatric disorder.[31] At least in such terrorists, ideology alone is not a sufficient explanation for injuring or killing others—abnormal brain function is a very likely root cause.

Brain Imaging Studies in Violent Individuals

While there are to our knowledge (aside from the three exceptions reported above) no direct neuropathological or imaging investigations of the brains of terrorists or persons running amok, numerous structural and functional brain-imaging studies have meanwhile been performed in violent criminal offenders and in persons with antisocial personality disorder (APD) with/ without psychopathy, a significant proportion of whom may be encountered among terrorists. The following sections provide an overview of the structural (see Table 8.1) and functional (see Table 8.2) imaging studies that investigated male adult violent samples published during the previous 10 years only (2008 to February of 2017). For earlier reviews, see, for example, Bufkin and Luttrell,[32] Raine et al.,[33] and Weber et al.[34]

Table 8.1 Structural imaging of aggression and violent behavior (studies investigating adult male samples with a history of violence, published between 2008 and 2017, in order by descending date)

Authors	Methods	Participants	Results
Leutgeb et al. (2016)[84]	MRI (VBM, ROI)	31 violent prisoners, 30 healthy controls	Prisoners vs. controls: GM volume cerebellum↑
Del Bene et al. (2016)[81]	MRI (ROI, whole-brain and ventricular volume)	37 violent and 26 nonviolent patients with schizophrenia, 24 nonpsychotic violent subjects, 24 healthy controls	Interaction effect violence & diagnosis in left AMY, violent nonpsychotic subjects: AMY↓ (potentially mediated by substance abuse)
Leutgeb et al. (2015)[43]	MRI (VBM)	40 violent offenders, 37 healthy controls	Offenders vs. controls: GM volume PFC↓, cerebellum↑, and basal ganglia↑
Pardini et al. (2014)[80]	MRI (ROI: AMY)	20 subjects with a history of chronic serious violence, 16 with transient serious violence, 20 without serious violence	Lower AMY volume associated with aggression, violence and psychopathic traits

Table 8.1 (cont.)

Authors	Methods	Participants	Results
Cope et al. (2014)[67]	MRI (VBM, whole-brain)	20 incarcerated who committed homicide, 135 other incarcerated	Homicide vs. no homicide: GM volume medial/lateral temporal lobe↓ (hippocampus, posterior insula)
Schiltz et al. (2013)[35]	MRI, computed tomography	162 violent and 125 nonviolent prison inmates, 52 noncriminal controls	Violent offenders > nonviolent offenders / noncriminal controls: morphological abnormalities (frontal/parietal and medial temporal structures, 3rd ventricle, left lateral ventricle)
Bertsch et al. (2013)[45]	MRI (VBM, ROI)	25 antisocial offenders (12 with borderline personality disorder, 13 with high psychopathic traits), 14 healthy noncriminals	Offenders with psychopathy vs. controls: GM volume left postcentral gyrus↓, left dorsal medial PFC↓, right posterior cingulate cortex/precuneus↓, occipital↓
Ly et al. (2012)[57]	MRI (cortical thickness)	21 psychopathic and 31 nonpsychopathic inmates	Psychopaths vs. nonpsychopaths: thinner left insula, left dorsal anterior cingulate cortex, precentral gyrus, temporal pole and right inferior frontal gyrus
Howner et al. (2012)[66]	MRI (cortical thickness)	7 offenders with psychopathy, 7 offenders with autism spectrum disorder, 12 healthy noncriminals	Psychopathic offenders vs. controls: thinner cortex in the temporal lobe and whole right hemisphere
Gregory (2012)[42]	MRI (VBM)	44 violent offenders with antisocial personality disorder (17 with and 27 without psychopathy), 22 healthy nonoffenders	Antisocial with vs. without psychopathy: GM volume anterior rostral PFC↓ and temporal pole↓
Ermer et al. (2012)[54]	MRI (VBM)	254 incarcerated men	Psychopathy: GM volume/concentration (para-) limbic areas↓ (parahippocampus, AMY, hippocampus, temporal pole, posterior cingulate cortex, OFC)

Table 8.1 (cont.)

Authors	Methods	Participants	Results
Cope et al. (2012)[56]	MRI (VBM, whole-brain)	66 participants (corrections centers)	Psychopathy: GM volume right insula↓, right hippocampus↓, OFC↑ and right anterior cingulate cortex↑
Schiffer et al. (2011)[73]	MRI (VBM)	24 violent offenders (12 with and 12 without substance use disorder), 13 nonoffenders with substance use disorder, 14 healthy controls	Violent offenders vs. nonoffenders: GM volume AMY↑, left nucleus accumbens↑, right caudate↑, left insula↓
Motzkin et al. (2011)[82]	MRI, diffusion tensor imaging (ROI: PFC)	14 psychopathic and 13 nonpsychopathic inmates	Psychopathy: structural integrity in right uncinate fasciculus↓
Boccardi et al. (2011)[55]	MRI	26 violent offenders with psychopathy, 25 healthy controls	Offenders vs. controls: GM density 20%↓ in OFC and midline structures; 30%↓ in basolateral nucleus; 10–30%↑ in central and lateral nuclei
Yang et al, (2010)[68]	MRI (ROI)	40 murderers (22 with and 18 without schizophrenia), 19 nonviolent patients with schizophrenia, 33 healthy controls	Murderers with schizophrenia vs. controls: GM volume hippocampus↓. Murderers without schizophrenia vs. controls: GM volume parahippocampus↓
Yang et al. (2010)[51]	MRI (ROI: AMY)	16 unsuccessful psychopaths, 10 successful psychopaths, 27 controls	Unsuccessful psychopaths vs. controls: GM volume middle frontal lobe↓, OFC↓, and AMY↓
Boccardi et al. (2010)[71]	MRI (ROI: hippocampus)	26 violent offenders with psychopathy (psychopathy scores: 12 high, 14 medium), 25 healthy controls	High vs. medium / controls: significant depression along longitudinal hippocampal axis; high/medium vs. controls: abnormal enlargement of lateral borders in both hippocampi

Table 8.1 (cont.)

Authors	Methods	Participants	Results
Kumari et al. (2009)[52]	MRI (ROI: PFC, temporal lobe, hippocampus, AMY)	10 violent and 14 nonviolent patients with schizophrenia, 14 healthy controls	Violent schizophrenic: impulsiveness↑, GM volume OFC↓, and hippocampus↓
Craig et al. (2009)[83]	Diffusion tensor imaging (ROI: AMY–OFC network)	9 inpatients with psychopathy, 9 healthy controls	Psychopaths vs. controls: fractional anisotropy in uncinate fasciculus↓
Tiihonen et al. (2008)[53]	MRI (VBM)	26 violent offenders (antisocial personality disorder, substance dependence), 25 healthy controls	Offenders vs. controls: white matter volume occipital↑, parietal↑, and left cerebellum↑, GM volume right cerebellum↑, atrophy in postcentral gyri, frontopolar cortex, and OFC
Puri et al. (2008)[69]	MRI (VBM, whole-brain)	13 violent and 13 nonviolent patients with schizophrenia	Violent vs. nonviolent: GM volume cerebellum↓, angular gyrus↓, and supramarginal gyrus↓
Müller et al. (2008)[41]	MRI (VBM, whole-brain)	17 forensic inpatients, 17 healthy controls	Inpatients vs. controls: GM volume reduction in temporal and frontal lobes, especially right superior temporal gyrus↓

AMY = amygdala; GM = gray matter; MRI = magnetic resonance imaging; OFC = orbitofrontal cortex; PFC = prefrontal cortex; ROI = region of interest; VBM = voxel-based morphometry.

Structural Imaging Findings (CT and MRI)

A more global assessment of brain pathology in violent persons was performed in a retrospective investigation by Schiltz and colleagues,[35] who qualitatively rated brain tissue defects in magnetic resonance imaging (MRI) and computed tomography (CT) scans from a large sample of incarcerated violent offenders in comparison to nonviolent offenders and nonoffending healthy controls. Violent offenders compared to the two nonoffender groups displayed a considerable higher rate of brain abnormalities. The observed brain damage or atrophy was located mainly in the frontal and medial temporal brain regions.[35]

Table 8.2 Studies of functional imaging of aggressive and violent behavior (studies investigating adult male samples with a history of violence, published between 2008 and 2017, in order of descending date)

Authors	Methods	Participants	Results
Leutgeb et al. (2016)[84]	fMRI	31 criminal prisoners, 30 noncriminal controls	Criminals: functional connectivity ↑ between left AMY and right cerebellum, functional connectivity ↓ between OFC and cerebellum, functional connectivity ↑ within dorsolateral PFC
Contreras-Rodríguez et al. (2015)[96]	fMRI	22 criminal psychopaths, 22 noncriminal controls	Psychopaths: functional connectivity ↑ within dorsomedial frontal cortex, functional connectivity ↓ between PFC and AMY, hippocampus
Decety et al. (2014)[104]	fMRI	27 incarcerated high-psychopaths, 28 incarcerated medium-psychopaths, 25 incarcerated low-psychopaths	Dysfunction in face processing in high-psychopathic offenders: frontal activity (OFC, ventromedial PFC, inferior frontal gyrus) ↓, activity in the fusiform gyrus ↓
Mier et al. (2014)[93]	fMRI	11 imprisoned psychopaths, 18 healthy controls	Dysfunction in face processing in psychopathic inmates: activation ↓ in fusiform gyrus Dysfunction in theory of mind in psychopathic inmates: activation ↓ in AMY and inferior frontal gyrus
Decety et al. (2013)[92]	fMRI	27 incarcerated high-psychopaths, 28 incarcerated medium-psychopaths, 25 incarcerated low-psychopaths	Empathy dysfunction in high-psychopathic inmates: activation ↓ in ventromedial PFC and lateral OFC whereas activation ↑ in insula
Decety et al. (2013)[99]	fMRI	37 incarcerated high-psychopaths, 44 incarcerated medium-psychopaths, 40 incarcerated low-psychopaths	Empathy dysfunction in high-psychopathic inmates: functional connectivity ↓ between anterior insula and AMY with OFC and ventromedial PFC

Table 8.2 (cont.)

Authors	Methods	Participants	Results
Meffert et al. (2013)[101]	fMRI	18 psychopathic offenders, 26 controls	In psychopaths, brain regions for empathy were not spontaneously activated when participants were instructed to feel with the actors
Prehn et al. (2013)[105]	fMRI	15 offenders with borderline and antisocial personality disorder, 17 healthy controls	Reactivity ↑ of the left AMY in offenders
Pujara et al. (2013)[106]	fMRI	18 incarcerated psychopaths, 23 incarcerated nonpsychopaths	The more psychopathic, activation ↑ in the left ventral striatum
Pujol et al. (2012)[100]	fMRI	22 criminal psychopaths, 22 noncriminal controls	Moral judgment dysfunction in criminal psychopaths: activation ↓ in medial frontal cortices, posterior cingulate cortex and hippocampus. Functional connectivity ↓ between medial frontal cortices and posterior cingulate cortex
Ly et al. (2012)[57]	fMRI	20 psychopathic inmates, 20 non-psychopathic inmates	Psychopathic inmates: functional connectivity ↓ between left insula and left dorsal anterior cingulate cortex
Harenski et al. (2010)[98]	fMRI	16 incarcerated psychopaths, 16 incarcerated nonpsychopaths	Moral judgment dysfunction in incarcerated psychopaths: activation ↓ in ventromedial PFC and anterior temporal cortex
Sommer et al. (2010)[107]	fMRI	14 criminal psychopathic patients, 14 criminal nonpsychopathic patients	Empathy dysfunction in criminal psychopaths: activation ↑ in OFC, medial frontal cortices and temporoparietal areas
Dolan & Fullam (2009)[108]	fMRI	12 low-psychopathic schizophrenia violent offenders, 12 high-psychopathic schizophrenia violent offenders	The more psychopathic, activation ↓ in the AMY

Table 8.2 (cont.)

Authors	Methods	Participants	Results
Kumari et al. (2009)[109]	fMRI	14 nonviolent healthy controls, 13 schizophrenia and violence, 13 schizophrenia without violence, 13 with antisocial personality disorder and violence	Threat anticipation dysfunction in violent people: thalamic–striatal activity↑ in schizophrenia, thalamic–striatal activity↓ in antisocial personality disorder
Yang & Raine (2009)[95]	fMRI, PET, SPECT, MRS	31 functional studies (and 12 structural studies)	Prefrontal functioning↓ (right OFC, left dorsolateral PFC, right anterior cingulate cortex) in antisocial individuals
Lee et al. (2008)[97]	fMRI	10 batterers, 13 controls	Batterers: limbic activation↑ and frontal activation↓ to aggressive stimuli
Lee et al. (2008)[103]	fMRI	10 batterers, 13 controls	Batterers: responsivity↑, e.g., in hippocampus to threat stimuli

AMY = amygdala; fMRI = functional magnetic resonance imaging; MRS = magnetic resonance spectroscopy; OFC = orbitofrontal cortex; PET = positron emission tomography; PFC = prefrontal cortex; SPECT = single-photon emission computed tomography.

Frontal Lobe and Violence

Frontal cortical pathology seems to play a major role in the pathophysiology of violent behavior. The frontal cortex is an anatomically and functionally heterogeneous brain structure involved, for example, in executive functioning, motor control, behavioral/emotional self-regulation, social behavior, and moral decision making.[36–39] Frontal lobe abnormalities have been found consistently in morphometric neuroimaging studies.[40,41] Prefrontal cortex (PFC) abnormalities especially seem to be involved in aggressive and violent behavior.[42,43] There is an association between prefrontal volume reduction and aggression as well as antisocial behavior. This is also evident in subjects with both traumatic and neurodegenerative impairments of the prefrontal areas.[40] PFC involvement in executive functioning could further be associated with deficits in decision making as well as problems in behavioral control.[44] When comparing violent offenders with APD and psychopathy to violent offenders with APD but without psychopathy, a reduced amount of gray matter (GM) was found bilaterally in the anterior rostral medial

PFC.[42] Moreover, in antisocial offenders with high-psychopathic traits there was a significant volume reduction in the dorsomedial PFC.[45]

One part of the prefrontal cortex, the orbitofrontal cortex (OFC), is relevant for processing of reward/punishment, emotion regulation, self-control, and behavioral inhibition,[46–48] and is interconnected with the limbic areas.[49] Specifically, OFC lesions are associated with an increase in aggression and impulsiveness, socially inadequate behavior, and enhanced disinhibition.[40,50] It is a quite consistent finding that the orbitofrontal GM volume is reduced in male adult samples inclined to violence. OFC tissue reductions have been reported in unsuccessful psychopaths (prosecuted for their violent crimes) as compared to successful psychopaths (not prosecuted),[51] but also in violent patients with schizophrenia,[52] as well as in violent offenders with APD as compared to healthy controls.[53] Aside from volume reductions, a decreased orbitofrontal GM concentration was found in incarcerated men with psychopathy,[54] and a 20 per cent reduced GM density was reported in the OFC and frontal midline structures when comparing violent offenders with psychopathic and healthy controls.[55] However, there is also one study that reported an increased orbitofrontal GM volume in inmates with psychopathy.[56]

Another focus of structural findings is the anterior cingulate cortex, which is situated beside the midline and is involved in the emotion-regulation circuitry. Abnormalities in this area are associated with an increased propensity for violent behavior[46] and/or with psychopathy as compared to nonpsychopathic inmates.[57] The posterior cingulate cortex is found to be impaired in persons inclined to violence, too. This brain area is linked to cognitive functions, including regulating attentional focus, and belongs to the so-called default mode network.[58–60] In incarcerated men, psychopathy was associated with GM volume and concentration reductions in the posterior cingulate cortex.[54] Furthermore, this region was smaller in another investigation of violent offenders versus healthy nonviolent controls.[53] An atrophy was also reported in the frontopolar cortex.[53] The right inferior frontal gyrus was found to be thinner in psychopathic versus nonpsychopathic inmates.[57] The posterior part of this gyrus, the pars opercularis, belongs to the mirror neuron system and is involved in imitation as well as social reciprocity.[61]

Temporal Lobe

The many functions of the temporal lobe involve emotional and social processes, including theory of mind, meaning the ability to recognize the thoughts and feelings of others, and to empathize.[37] Many studies have shown that temporal lobe damage can cause aggressive and violent behavior.[62] For example, in patients with temporal lobe epilepsy, a high incidence of behavior comparable to psychopathic habits was described—for example, hostility, diminished empathy, and even aggressive outbursts.[63] Furthermore, antisocial and socially inappropriate behavior were found to be associated with temporal brain alterations in frontotemporal dementia.[64,65]

The temporal cortex was found to be thinner in offenders with psychopathy when compared with healthy noncriminals.[66] Furthermore, the temporal gray matter volume was reduced in forensic inpatients compared to healthy controls.[41] In particular, the medial and lateral temporal regions were reported to have gray matter loss in incarcerated men who committed homicide compared to other crimes.[67]

Hippocampal Formation, Parahippocampal Gyrus

Reduced GM volume and concentration in the hippocampal formation was found to occur in criminal psychopathy.[54] A decreased hippocampal and parahippocampal volume was further described in a study comparing murderers with schizophrenia to nonschizophrenic murderers.[68] This is in line with findings of a reduced volume of the parahippocampal gyrus in violent offenders compared to healthy men.[53] Hippocampal tissue was found to be reduced bilaterally in incarcerated men who committed homicide compared to men sentenced for other crimes,[67] but also in incarcerated men with psychopathy,[54,56] as well as in violent patients with schizophrenia.[69] There are reports of increased impulsiveness in patients with schizophrenia inclined to repetitive violence, which was associated with reduced hippocampal volume.[52] When comparing high Psychopathy Checklist–Revised (PCL–R[70]) scorers with medium PCL–R scorers or healthy controls, a significant reduction along the hippocampal axis was described.[71]

The insula also belongs to the brain system involved in emotional experiences and empathy.[72] The left insular cortex was reported to be thinner in psychopathic versus nonpsychopathic inmates.[57] The left insular cortical tissue was also found to be reduced in violent offenders compared to nonoffenders,[73] whereas inmates with psychopathy had a smaller right insular GM volume in another study.[56] A third study reported insular GM volume reductions: incarcerated men who committed homicide in comparison to inmates sentenced for other crimes had decreased cortical tissue in the posterior insula.[67]

With regard to the pole of the temporal lobe, another paralimbic area, aggression and violent behavior are also associated with cortical thinning and volume reduction. Psychopathic compared to nonpsychopathic inmates had thinner bilateral temporal poles.[57] In addition, psychopathy was associated with reduced temporal pole GM volume in two studies, one comparing antisocial personality-disordered violent offenders with and without psychopathy[42] and the other investigating incarcerated men with different PCL–R scores.[54] The latter study also reported temporal pole GM concentration reductions in psychopaths.[54] Cortical thinning has also been reported in the superior temporal gyrus.[57]

Amygdala

The amygdala is one of the key structures in recent neurobiological models of violence.[74] This medial temporal lobe structure is the central part of the limbic system and can be divided into three nuclear complexes: basolateral, centromedial, and cortical/superficial.[75,76] The amygdala is involved in fear conditioning, emotion expression and recognition, emotionally influenced memory, and moral reasoning.[75,77–79] Furthermore, it is a key structure for emotion regulation belonging to a circuitry that also consists of the orbital brain, the dorsolateral prefrontal cortex, and the anterior cingulate cortex.[46] Amygdala impairments have been linked to a variety of psychiatric disorders characterized by aggressive behavior (e.g., psychopathy and antisocial personality disorder). Psychopathy has been found to be associated with reduced amygdala GM volume in a sample of 254 incarcerated men.[54] Significantly reduced GM volume and cortical thickness of the amygdala were described in unsuccessful psychopaths compared to controls as well.[51] The three subnuclei are obviously associated with different structural amygdala impairments: in offenders with psychopathy, there was up to 30 per cent reduced brain tissue in the basolateral nucleus, and the central and lateral nuclei tissue were enlarged by 10 to 30 per cent.[55] Reduced amygdala volume seems to be associated with aggression and violence in general.[80] In violent but nonpsychotic subjects, violence was associated with volume reduction only in the left amygdala.[81] However, there is also one study that reported increased amygdala volume in violent offenders.[73]

In psychopathic individuals, the white matter connection between the amygdala and frontal brain areas (e.g., ventromedial PFC[82] and OFC[83]) is also impaired. There is an association between psychopathy and reduced structural integrity in the right uncinate fasciculus (connection from ventromedial PFC to amygdala), which is important for aggression and emotion regulation.[82] Furthermore, fractional anisotropy has been found to be reduced in the uncinated fasciculus in psychopaths compared to controls, suggesting an abnormal connection between the amygdala and the OFC.[83]

Further Brain Regions

Some studies have reported that the volume of the cerebellum is increased in violent offenders compared to healthy controls.[43,84] Aside from its main function of extrapyramidal motor coordination, the cerebellum is also involved in cognition and emotion as well as empathy (for pain) and moral judgments.[85–87] It is anatomically connected with brain regions associated with emotion regulation, aggression, and moral decisions, like the amygdala, the hippocampus, and the PFC.[88,89] However, one study found that cerebellar GM volume was reduced in violent patients with schizophrenia.[69] The cerebellum as well as the basal ganglia are relevant for motor aspects of impulsive acts.[90] The findings for the basal ganglia, however, are more inconsistent. There are reports of increased as well as decreased gray matter volumes of the caudate, putamen, pallidum, and nucleus accumbens in violent,[43,73] impulsive, or sensation-seeking[91] individuals. A few studies also found tissue reduction in the postcentral gyrus (lateral parietal lobe) in violent offenders or persons with psychopathic traits.[45,53] When comparing violent and nonviolent patients with schizophrenia, reduced GM volume in the angular gyrus (anterolateral parietal lobe)[69] as well as in the supramarginal gyrus (parietal lobe) has been found.[69]

Functional Imaging Studies in Violent Individuals

Frontal Lobe

In addition to the structural deficits found in subregions of the frontal lobe, many functional imaging studies have described frontal lobe dysfunctions in violent individuals. The lateral OFC of incarcerated psychopaths has been shown to be less activated by an empathy task.[92] In addition, the inferior frontal gyrus of imprisoned psychopaths is less activated by a theory-of-mind task.[93] There is already some evidence that subjects show different functional responses in their emotional empathy while watching computer-generated actors compared to actors in live-action movies.[94] A meta-analysis consisting of 31 functional (and 12 structural) studies[95] found that antisocial individuals have functional deficits in the right orbitofrontal, the left dorsolateral prefrontal cortex, and the right anterior cingulate cortex, and this effect persisted regardless of whether the subjects had to perform a cognitive or emotional task.

There is an impaired functional connectivity between the orbital brain and other brain areas. Criminal prisoners showed less functional connectivity between the orbital cortex and cerebellum,[96] and incarcerated psychopaths had less functional connectivity to the amygdala and the anterior insula.[92]

In the medial frontal cortex, criminal psychopaths showed decreased activation during performance of a moral-dilemma task.[57] Spousal abusers showed less activation in the left medial frontal cortex during threat stimuli.[97] Criminal psychopaths showed increased functional connectivity within the dorsomedial frontal cortex but less gray matter volume in the PFC, in contrast to nonoffender controls.[96] Reduced activation in the ventromedial PFC was found in incarcerated psychopaths during empathizing[92] as well as during a moral judgment task.[98]

Limbic Areas: Amygdala, Hippocampus, Cingulate Cortex

Reduced functional connectivity between the PFC and the limbic (amygdala, hippocampus) as well as paralimbic areas was found in criminal psychopaths.[96] Imprisoned psychopaths had increased activation in the amygdala when they performed a theory-of-mind task, and functional connectivity between the amygdala and the superior temporal gyrus was impaired.[93] When psychopathic offenders had to perform an empathy task with people in pain, activation in the amygdala correlated negatively with factor 1 of the PCL–R scale.[70] Factor 1 consists of the interpersonal facet (e.g., superficial charm or manipulative behavior) and the affective facet (e.g., callousness). The more interpersonal and affective deficits the subjects had, the less activation of the amygdala was found.[99] In nonpsychopathic offenders, a positive correlation between activation in the right amygdala and severity of moral judgment ratings was found. This implies that the higher activation in the right amygdala, the higher the severity of moral violation was rated, and this correlation was not found in psychopathic offenders.[98] In a cognitive control paradigm, spousal abusers showed increased activation of the right amygdala as well as of the hippocampus.[97] In contrast, the hippocampus was less activated in criminal psychopaths during a moral-dilemma task.[100]

Functional deficits in the cingulate cortex have also been found in violent offenders. Activation in the right anterior cingulate cortex was reduced in a cognitive control paradigm[97] and during empathizing.[101] The meta-analysis of Yang and Raine[95] showed that antisocial individuals have functional deficits in the right anterior cingulate cortex regardless of whether the subjects had to perform a cognitive or emotional task. Interestingly, activation in the right anterior cingulate cortex during empathizing increased after offenders were instructed to empathize with the actors.[101] The anterior cingulate cortex as well as the anterior insula belong to the empathy-for-pain network,[102] which is obviously dysfunctional in psychopathic criminals. Activation of the posterior cingulate cortex decreased in moral decision making[100] but increased after presenting threat stimuli.[103] The functional connectivity between the left dorsal anterior cingulate cortex and the left insula was reduced,[57] as well as the functional connectivity between the medial frontal cortex and the posterior cingulate cortex.[100]

Other Brain Areas

Several studies have shown functional deficits during face processing in the fusiform gyrus in criminal offenders: either a bilateral decreased activation in the fusiform gyrus in incarcerated psychopaths[93,104] or reduced activation only in the left fusiform gyrus in spousal abusers incarcerated because of domestic violence.[97]

Activation in the insula of high-psychopathic inmates was increased during empathizing.[92] Conversely, the more interpersonal and affective deficits the psychopathic inmates had (measured by factor 1 of the PCL–R), the less activation in the insula.[99] Psychopathic offenders did not activate the insula spontaneously for vicarious pain representations, but, interestingly, activation in the insula increased after psychopaths were instructed to empathize with the actors.[101]

The more psychopathic the inmates, the higher the activation in the left ventral striatum (which belongs to the reward systems in the brain) when receiving monetary rewards. Furthermore, the greater the interpersonal and affective deficits of high-psychopathic offenders (measured with factor 1 of the PCL–R), the higher the activation of the ventral striatum during empathizing with other people who are in pain.[99]

Conclusions

In the search for neurobiological correlates, aggressive and violent behaviors are usually subdivided into an impulsive/reactive subtype (aggressive rage) and an instrumental/proactive subtype (predatory attack). For the human spectrum of aggressive behavior, however, there is no strict subdivision in a categorical sense of these two types of violence; rather, they reflect a continuum with a broadly overlapping symptomatology between the two poles.[23]

As initially shown in this article, there is evidence from brain stimulation studies in experimental animals, as well as from stereotactic stimulations in humans, that different neuronal cell groups in the hypothalamus and amygdala can be regarded as phylogenetically very old "neuronal generators" of these different poles of aggression, which are controlled by inhibiting or activating fibers from the cortical, limbic, and paralimbic brain regions.

With regard to the possible neurobiological substrates of terrorism, the instrumental/proactive subtype, which can be encountered in many criminal offenders with psychopathy, seems to be more applicable to terrorists than the impulsive subtype. The latter might be more prevalent in persons running amok or in offenders who commit manslaughter in the heat of the moment.

Despite some inconsistencies due to methodological or sample differences, the structural and functional imaging studies in adult male samples with a history of violence reviewed here over the previous 10 years give the following general (statistical) pattern for brain dysfunctions for the two subtypes (poles) of violent individuals:

Impulsive/reactive violence: reduced volume in prefrontal, orbitofrontal and mesiotemporal structures (hippocampus, parahippocampus); diminished frontal activation and functional connectivity but increased limbic hippocampal and amygdala reactivity (depending on the activation paradigm).

Instrumental/proactive violence (mainly associated with psychopathy): decreased gray matter of orbitofrontal and prefrontal cortex, deceased volume of all temporolimbic structures (amygdala, hippocampus, parahippocampal gyrus) as well as of the insular cortex; reduced functional activation of the frontal and temporolimbic (amygdala, hippocampus, temporal pole, fusiform gyrus) and posterior cingulate cortex; diminished functional connectivity between the frontal cortical regions (orbitofrontal, ventromedial prefrontal, inferior frontal gyrus) with the limbic areas (amygdala, hippocampus), anterior insula, and posterior cingulate cortex.

To the best of our knowledge, there have been no imaging studies of the very small hypothalamic group of neurons that produce aggression by direct stimulation, because it is much more difficult to localize and delineate them accurately, even with the best available high-resolution imaging techniques. However, it is clear that the cortical regions essentially located at the basal frontal and medial temporal lobe projecting to the amygdala and thereby controlling aggression generating limbic and diencephalic networks show structural and functional defects in impulsive violent men. On the other hand, there is an impressive overlap between the regional pattern of structural and functional deficits in violent offenders of the psychopathic type with the brain regions that are crucial in the neuronal networks for empathy and compassion. These brain areas are involved in the vicarious suffering for unpleasant feelings like the pain of others (empathy) and for positive devotion and care for others, as well as a motivation to improve the other's well-being (compassion).[102] There is no doubt that such individuals are overrepresented among terrorists. The malfunctioning brain areas in psychopaths involve the inferior frontal, subgenual, anterior insular, and cingulate cortex.

In addition, many terrorists might have feelings of superiority, dominance, and satisfaction when performing terroristic attacks, suggesting that a hedonistic component via activation of reward systems in the brain plays an additional role, especially during collective violent acts. However, as far as we know, as yet no functional imaging studies of brain reward structure systems in violent psychopathic perpetrators are available.

The present debate on the causes of terrorism is still dominated by social, psychodynamic, political, and economic arguments and perspectives, and, indeed, it seems plausible that under peculiar psychosocial conditions even normal people with no previous signs of psychopathology become willing to perform cruelties against others.[24–29] However, our knowledge of the neurobiological basis of violence as well as the reported brain-imaging findings should enrich this debate by also taking aspects of brain pathology into account.

Disclosures

Bernhard Bogerts, Maria Schöne, and Stephanie Breitschuh hereby declare that they have nothing to disclose.

References

1. Bogerts, B. Gehirn und Verbrechen: Neurobiologie von Gewalttaten. In: Schneider F, ed. *Entwicklungen der Psychiatrie*. Berlin, Heidelberg: Springer; 2006: 335–347.

2. Report to the Governor, Medical Aspects, Charles J. Whitman Catastrophe. Austin: The Whitman Archives; 1966. http://alt.cimedia.com/statesman/specialreports/whitman/findings.pdf. Accessed July 6, 2017.

3. Eagleman, D. The brain on trial. Atl Mon. July/August 2011. www.theatlantic.com/magazine/archive/2011/07/the-brain-on-trial/308520/. Accessed July 6, 2017.

4. MacLean, PD. Some psychiatric implications of physiological studies on fronto-temporal portion of limbic system (visceral brain). *Electroencephalogr Clin Neurophysiol*. 1952; 4(4): 407–418.

5. Hess, WR. *Das Zwischenhirn: Syndrome, Lokalisationen, Funktionen*. Basel: Schwabe; 1949.

6. Wasman, M, Flynn, JP. Directed attack elicited from the hypothalamus. *Arch Neurol*. 1962; 6: 220–227.

7. Ploog, D. Biologische Grundlagen aggressiven Verhaltens: Psychiatrische und ethologische Aspekte abnormen Verhaltens [in German]. In: Kranz H, Heinrich K, eds. *Erste Düsseldorfer Symposium*. Stuttgart: Thieme; 1974: 49–77.

8. Bogerts, B, Möller-Leimkühler, AM. Neurobiologische Ursachen und psychosoziale Bedingungen individueller Gewalt [Neurobiological and psychosocial causes of individual male violence] [in German]. *Nervenarzt*. 2013; 84(11): 1329–1344.

9. Mark, VH, Erwin, FR. *Violence and the Brain*. New York, NY: Harper & Row; 1970.

10. Klüver, H, Bucy, PC. "Psychic blindness" and other symptoms following bilateral temporal lobectomy in rhesus monkeys. *Am J Physiol*. 1937; 119: 352–353.

11. Bogerts, B. The temporolimbic system theory of positive schizophrenic symptoms. *Schizophr Bull*. 1997; 23(3): 423–436.

12. Bogerts, B. The neuropathology of schizophrenic diseases: historical aspects and present knowledge. *Eur Arch Psychiatry Clin Neurosci*. 1999; 249(Suppl 4): 2–13.

13. Fazel, S, Gulati, G, Linsell, L, Geddes, JR, Grann, M. Schizophrenia and violence: systematic review and meta-analysis. *PLoS Med*. 2009; 6(8): e1000120. www.ncbi.nlm.nih.gov/pmc/articles/PMC2718581/. Accessed July 6, 2017.

14. Gómez, JM, Verdú, M, González-Megías, A, Méndez, M. The phylogenetic roots of human lethal violence. *Nature*. 2016; 538(7624): 233–237.

15. Choi, JK, Bowles, S. The coevolution of parochial altruism and war. *Science*. 2007; **318**(5850): 636–640.

16. Jung, H, Herrenkohl, TI, Lee, JO, Klika, JB, Skinner, ML. Effects of physical and emotional child abuse and its chronicity on crime into adulthood. *Violence Vict.* 2015; **30**(6): 1004–1018.

17. DiLalla, DL, Carey, G, Gottesman, II, Bouchard, TJ, Jr. Heritability of MMPI personality indicators of psychopathology in twins reared apart. *J Abnorm Psychol.* 1996; **105**(4): 491–499.

18. Joyal, CC, Putkonen, A, Mancini-Marïe, A, et al. Violent persons with schizophrenia and comorbid disorders: a functional magnetic resonance imaging study. *Schizophr Res.* 2007; **91**(1–3): 97–102.

19. Rhee, SH, Waldman, ID. Genetic and environmental influences on antisocial behavior: a meta-analysis of twin and adoption studies. *Psychol Bull.* 2002; **128**(3): 490–529.

20. Alia-Klein, N, Goldstein, RZ, Kriplani, A, et al. Brain monoamine oxidase A activity predicts trait aggression. *J Neurosci.* 2008; **28**(19): 5099–5104.

21. Buckholtz, JW, Meyer-Lindenberg, A. MAOA and the neurogenetic architecture of human aggression. *Trends Neurosci.* 2008; **31**(3): 120–129.

22. Caspi, A, Moffitt, TE. Gene–environment interactions in psychiatry: joining forces with neuroscience. *Nat Rev Neurosci.* 2006; **7**(7): 583–590.

23. Rosell, DR, Siever, LJ. The neurobiology of aggression and violence. *CNS Spectr.* 2015; **20**(3): 254–279.

24. Browning, CR. *Ordinary Men: Reserve Police Battalion 101 and the Final Solution in Poland*. New York, NY: HarperCollins and Aaron Asher Books; 1992.

25. Haney, C, Banks, C, Zimbardo, P. Interpersonal dynamics in a simulated prison. *Int J Criminology Penol.* 1973; 1: 69–97; http://pdf.prisonexp.org/ijcp1973.pdf. Accessed July 6, 2017.

26. Milgram, S. Behavioral study of obedience. *J Abnorm Psychol.* 1963; **67**(4): 371–378.

27. Milgram, S. *Obedience to Authority: An Experimental View*. New York, NY: Harper; 1974.

28. Zimbardo, P. *The Lucifer Effect: Understanding How Good People Turn Evil*. Random House Reprints; 2008.

29. Möller-Leimkühler, AM, Bogerts, B. Kollektive Gewalt [Collective violence: neurobiological, psychosocial and sociological condition] [in German]. *Nervenarzt.* 2013; **84**(11): 1345–1358.

30. Bundesamt für Verfassungsschutz. *Analyse der den deutschen Sicherheitsbehörden vorliegenden Informationen über die Radikalisierungshintergründe und -verläufe der Personen, die aus islamistischer Motivation aus Deutschland in Richtung Syrien*

ausgereist sind—so lautet der Titel [in German]; Ständige Konferenz der Innenminister und senatoren der Linder; 2016. www.innenministerkonferenz.de/ IMK/DE/termine/to-beschluesse/14–12-11_12/anlage-analyse.pdf?__blob=publica tionFile&v=2. Accessed July 6, 2017.

31. Pantucci, R, Ellis, C, Chaplais, L. *Lone-Actor Terrorism: Literature Review.* London: Royal United Service Institute; 2015.

32. Bufkin, JL, Luttrell, VR. Neuroimaging studies of aggressive and violent behavior: current findings and implications for criminology and criminal justice. *Trauma, Violence Abuse.* 2005; **6**(2): 176–191.

33. Raine, A, Yang, Y. Neural foundations to moral reasoning and antisocial behavior. *Soc Cogn Affect Neurosci.* 2006; **1**(3): 203–213.

34. Weber, S, Habel, U, Amunts, K, Schneider, F. Structural brain abnormalities in psychopaths: a review. *Behav Sci Law.* 2008; **26**(1): 7–28.

35. Schiltz, K, Witzel, JG, Bausch-Hölterhoff, J, Bogerts, B. High prevalence of brain pathology in violent prisoners: a qualitative CT and MRI scan study. *Eur Arch Psychiatry Clin Neurosci.* 2013; **263**(7): 607–616.

36. Floden, D. Frontal lobe function. In: Parsons MW, Hammeke TA, Snyder PJ, eds. *Clinical Neuropsychology: A Pocket Handbook for Assessment.* Washington, DC: American Psychological Association; 2014: 498–524.

37. Olson, IR, Plotzker, A, Ezzyat, Y. The enigmatic temporal pole: a review of findings on social and emotional processing. *Brain.* 2007; **130**(7): 1718–1731.

38. Rudebeck, PH, Bannerman, DM, Rushworth, MF. The contribution of distinct subregions of the ventromedial frontal cortex to emotion, social behavior, and decision making. *Cogn Affect Behav Neurosci.* 2008; **8**(4): 485–497.

39. Stuss, DT. Functions of the frontal lobes: relation to executive functions. *J Int Neuropsychol Soc.* 2011; **17**(5): 759–765.

40. Brower, MC, Price, BH. Neuropsychiatry of frontal lobe dysfunction in violent and criminal behaviour: a critical review. *J Neurol Neurosurg Psychiatry.* 2001; **71**(6): 720–726.

41. Müller, JL, Gänßbauer, S, Sommer, M, et al. Gray matter changes in right superior temporal gyrus in criminal psychopaths: evidence from voxel-based morphometry. *Psychiatry Res.* 2008; **163**(3): 213–222.

42. Gregory, S. The antisocial brain: psychopathy matters. *Arch Gen Psychiatry.* 2012; **69**(9): 962–972.

43. Leutgeb, V, Leitner, M, Wabnegger, A, et al. Brain abnormalities in high-risk violent offenders and their association with psychopathic traits and criminal recidivism. *Neuroscience.* 2015; **308**: 194–201.

44. Domenech, P, Koechlin, E. Executive control and decision-making in the prefrontal cortex. *Curr Opin Behav Sci.* 2015; **1**: 101–106.

45. Bertsch, K, Grothe, M, Prehn, K, et al. Brain volumes differ between diagnostic groups of violent criminal offenders. *Eur Arch Psychiatry Clin Neurosci*. 2013; **263** (7): 593–606.

46. Davidson, RJ. Dysfunction in the neural circuitry of emotion regulation: a possible prelude to violence. *Science*. 2000; **289**(5479): 591–594.

47. Kringelbach, ML, Rolls, ET. The functional neuroanatomy of the human orbito-frontal cortex: evidence from neuroimaging and neuropsychology. *Prog Neurobiol*. 2004; **72**(5): 341–372.

48. Rudebeck, PH, Murray, EA. The orbitofrontal oracle: cortical mechanisms for the prediction and evaluation of specific behavioral outcomes. *Neuron*. 2014; **84**(6): 1143–1156.

49. Schoenbaum, G, Roesch, MR, Stalnaker, TA. Orbitofrontal cortex, decision-making and drug addiction. *Trends Neurosci*. 2006; **29**(2): 116–124.

50. Birbaumer, N, Veit, R, Lotze, M, et al. Deficient fear conditioning in psychopathy: a functional magnetic resonance imaging study. *Arch Gen Psychiatry*. 2005; **62**(7): 799–805.

51. Yang, Y, Raine, A, Colletti, P, Toga, AW, Narr, KL. Morphological alterations in the prefrontal cortex and the amygdala in unsuccessful psychopaths. *J Abnorm Psychol*. 2010; **119**(3): 546–554.

52. Kumari, V, Barkataki, I, Goswami, S, Flora, S, Das, M, Taylor, P. Dysfunctional, but not functional, impulsivity is associated with a history of seriously violent behaviour and reduced orbitofrontal and hippocampal volumes in schizophrenia. *Psychiatry Res*. 2009; **173**(1): 39–44.

53. Tiihonen, J, Rossi, R, Laakso, MP, et al. Brain anatomy of persistent violent offenders: more rather than less. *Psychiatry Res*. 2008; **163**(3): 201–212.

54. Ermer, E, Cope, LM, Calhoun, VD, Nyalakanti, PK, Kiehl, KA. Aberrant paralimbic gray matter in criminal psychopathy. *J Abnorm Psychol*. 2012; **121**(3): 649–658.

55. Boccardi, M, Frisoni, GB, Hare, RD, et al. Cortex and amygdala morphology in psychopathy. *Psychiatry Res*. 2011; **193**(2): 85–92.

56. Cope, LM, Shane, MS, Segall, JM, et al. Examining the effect of psychopathic traits on gray matter volume in a community substance abuse sample. *Psychiatry Res*. 2012; **204**(2–3): 91–100.

57. Ly, M, Motzkin, JC, Philippi, CL, et al. Cortical thinning in psychopathy. *Am J Psychiatry*. 2012; **169**(7): 743–749.

58. Buckner, RL, Andrews-Hanna, JR, Schacter, DL. The brain's default network: anatomy, function, and relevance to disease. *Ann N Y Acad Sci*. 2008; **1124**: 1–38.

59. Hahn, B, Ross, TJ, Stein, EA. Cingulate activation increases dynamically with response speed under stimulus unpredictability. *Cereb Cortex*. 2007; **17**(7): 1664–1671.

60. Leech, R, Sharp, DJ. The role of the posterior cingulate cortex in cognition and disease. *Brain*. 2014; **137**(1): 12–32.

61. Yamasaki, S, Yamasue, H, Abe, O, et al. Reduced gray matter volume of pars opercularis is associated with impaired social communication in high-functioning autism spectrum disorders. *Biol Psychiatry*. 2010; **68**(12): 1141–1147.

62. Bannon, SM, Salis, KL, O'Leary, DK. Structural brain abnormalities in aggression and violent behavior. *Aggress Violent Behav*. 2015; **25**(Pt B): 323–331.

63. Kiehl, KA. A cognitive neuroscience perspective on psychopathy: evidence for paralimbic system dysfunction. *Psychiatry Res*. 2006; **142**(2–3): 107–128.

64. Miller, BL, Darby, A, Benson, DF, Cummings, JL, Miller, MH. Aggressive, socially disruptive and antisocial behaviour associated with fronto-temporal dementia. *Br J Psychiatry*. 1997; **170**(2): 150–154.

65. Woermann, FG, van Elst, LT, Koepp, MJ, et al. Reduction of frontal neocortical grey matter associated with an affective aggression in patients with temporal lobe epilepsy: an objective voxel-by-voxel analysis of automatically segmented MRI. *J Neurol Neurosurg Psychiatry*. 2000; **68**: 162–169.

66. Howner, K, Eskildsen, SF, Fischer, H, et al. Thinner cortex in the frontal lobes in mentally disordered offenders. *Psychiatry Res*. 2012; **203**(2–3): 126–131.

67. Cope, LM, Ermer, E, Gaudet, LM, et al. Abnormal brain structure in youth who commit homicide. *Neuroimage Clin*. 2014; **4**: 800–807.

68. Yang, Y, Raine, A, Han, CB, Schug, RA, Toga, AW, Narr, KL. Reduced hippocampal and parahippocampal volumes in murderers with schizophrenia. *Psychiatry Res*. 2010; **182**(1): 9–13.

69. Puri, BK, Counsell, SJ, Saeed, N, Bustos, MG, Treasaden, IH, Bydder, GM. Regional grey matter volumetric changes in forensic schizophrenia patients: an MRI study comparing the brain structure of patients who have seriously and violently offended with that of patients who have not. *BMC Psychiatry*. 2008; **8**(Suppl 1): S6.

70. Hare, RD. *The Hare Psychopathy Checklist–Revised (PCL–R)*. Toronto: Multi-Health Systems; 1991.

71. Boccardi, M, Ganzola, R, Rossi, R, et al. Abnormal hippocampal shape in offenders with psychopathy. *Hum Brain Mapp*. 2010; **31**(3): 438–447.

72. Eres, R, Decety, J, Louis, WR, Molenberghs, P. Individual differences in local gray matter density are associated with differences in affective and cognitive empathy. *Neuroimage*. 2015; **117**: 305–310.

73. Schiffer, B, Mueller, BW, Scherbaum, N, et al. Disentangling structural brain alterations associated with violent behavior from those associated with substance use disorders. *Arch Gen Psychiatry*. 2011; **68**(10): 1039–1049.

74. Siever, LJ. Neurobiology of aggression and violence. *Am J Psychiatry*. 2008; **165**(4): 429–442.

75. Price, JL. Amygdala. In: Squire LR, ed. *New Encyclopedia of Neuroscience*. New York, NY: Academic Press; 2008: 1–4.

76. Sah, P, Faber, ES, Lopez De Armentia, M, Power, J. The amygdaloid complex: anatomy and physiology. *Physiol Rev*. 2003; **83**(3): 803–834.

77. Blair, RJ. The amygdala and ventromedial prefrontal cortex in morality and psychopathy. *Trends Cogn Sci*. 2007; **11**(9): 387–392.

78. Phelps, EA. Human emotion and memory: interactions of the amygdala and hippocampal complex. *Curr Opin Neurobiol*. 2004; **14**(2): 198–202.

79. Phillips, RG, LeDoux, JE. Differential contribution of amygdala and hippocampus to cued and contextual fear conditioning. *Behav Neurosci*. 1992; **106**(2): 274–285.

80. Pardini, DA, Raine, A, Erickson, K, Loeber, R. Lower amygdala volume in men is associated with childhood aggression, early psychopathic traits, and future violence. *Biol Psychiatry*. 2014; **75**(1): 73–80.

81. Del Bene, VA, Foxe, JJ, Ross, LA, Krakowski, MI, Czobor, P, De Sanctis, P. Neuroanatomical abnormalities in violent individuals with and without a diagnosis of schizophrenia. *PLOS ONE*. 2016; 11(12):e0168100. www.ncbi.nlm.nih.gov/pmc/articles/PMC5193361/. Accessed July 6, 2017.

82. Motzkin, JC, Newman, JP, Kiehl, KA, Koenigs, M. Reduced prefrontal connectivity in psychopathy. *J Neurosci*. 2011; **31**(48): 17348–17357.

83. Craig, MC, Catani, M, Deeley, Q, et al. Altered connections on the road to psychopathy. *Mol Psychiatry*. 2009; **14**(10): 946–953; 907.

84. Leutgeb, V, Wabnegger, A, Leitner, M, et al. Altered cerebellar-amygdala connectivity in violent offenders: a resting-state fMRI study. *Neurosci Lett*. 2016; **610**: 160–164.

85. Harada, T, Itakura, S, Xu, F, et al. Neural correlates of the judgment of lying: a functional magnetic resonance imaging study. *Neurosci Res*. 2009; **63**(1): 24–34.

86. Lang, S, Yu, T, Markl, A, Müller, F, Kotchoubey, B. Hearing others' pain: neural activity related to empathy. *Cogn Affect Behav Neurosci*. 2011; **11**(3): 386–395.

87. Schmahmann, JD. Disorders of the cerebellum: ataxia, dysmetria of thought, and the cerebellar cognitive affective syndrome. *J Neuropsychiatry Clin Neurosci*. 2004; **16**(3): 367–378.

88. Demirtas-Tatlidede, A, Schmahmann, JD. Morality: incomplete without the cerebellum? *Brain*. 2013; **136**(8): 2007–2009.

89. Turner, BM, Paradiso, S, Marvel, CL, et al. The cerebellum and emotional experience. *Neuropsychologia*. 2007; **45**(6): 1331–1341.

90. Picazio, S, Koch, G. Is motor inhibition mediated by cerebello-cortical interactions? *Cerebellum*. 2015; **14**(1): 47–49.

91. Glenn, AL, Raine, A, Yaralian, PS, Yang, Y. Increased volume of the striatum in psychopathic individuals. *Biol Psychiatry*. 2010; **67**(1): 52–58.

92. Decety, J, Skelly, LR, Kiehl, KA. Brain response to empathy-eliciting scenarios involving pain in incarcerated psychopaths. *JAMA Psychiatry*. 2013; **70**(6): 638–645.

93. Mier, D, Haddad, L, Diers, K, Dressing, H, Meyer-Lindenberg, A, Kirsch, P. Reduced embodied simulation in psychopathy. *World J Biol Psychiatry*. 2014; **15** (6): 479–487.

94. Vemuri, K, Surampudi, BR. Evidence of stimulus correlated empathy modes: group ICA of fMRI data. *Brain Cogn*. 2015; **94**: 32–43.

95. Yang, Y, Raine, A. Prefrontal structural and functional brain imaging findings in antisocial, violent, and psychopathic individuals: a meta-analysis. *Psychiatry Res*. 2009; **174**(2): 81–88.

96. Contreras-Rodriguez, O, Pujol, J, Batalla, I, et al. Functional connectivity bias in the prefrontal cortex of psychopaths. *Biol Psychiatry*. 2015; **78**(9): 647–655.

97. Lee, TM, Chan, SC, Raine, A. Strong limbic and weak frontal activation to aggressive stimuli in spouse abusers. *Mol Psychiatry*. 2008; **13**(7): 655–656.

98. Harenski, CL, Harenski, KA, Shane, MS, Kiehl, KA. Aberrant neural processing of moral violations in criminal psychopaths. *J Abnorm Psychol*. 2010; **119**(4): 863–874.

99. Decety, J, Chen, C, Harenski, C, Kiehl, KA. An fMRI study of affective perspective taking in individuals with psychopathy: imagining another in pain does not evoke empathy. *Front Hum Neurosci*. 2013; **7**: 1–12.

100. Pujol, J, Batalla, I, Contreras-Rodríguez, O, et al. Breakdown in the brain network subserving moral judgment in criminal psychopathy. *Soc Cogn Affect Neurosci*. 2012; **7**(8): 917–923.

101. Meffert, H, Gazzola, V, den Boer, JA, Bartels, AA, Keysers, C. Reduced spontaneous but relatively normal deliberate vicarious representations in psychopathy. *Brain*. 2013; **136**(8): 2550–2562.

102. Singer, T, Klimecki, OM. Empathy and compassion. *Curr Biol*. 2014; **24**(18): R875–R878.

103. Lee, TM, Chan, SC, Raine, A. Hyperresponsivity to threat stimuli in domestic violence offenders: a functional magnetic resonance imaging study. *J Clin Psychiatry*. 2008; **70**(1): 36–45.

104. Decety, J, Skelly, L, Yoder, KJ, Kiehl, KA. Neural processing of dynamic emotional facial expressions in psychopaths. *Soc Neurosci*. 2014; **9**(1): 36–49.

105. Prehn, K, Schulze, L, Rossmann, S, et al. Effects of emotional stimuli on working memory processes in male criminal offenders with borderline and antisocial personality disorder. *World J Biol Psychiatry*. 2013; **14**(1): 71–78.

106. Pujara, M, Motzkin, JC, Newman, JP, Kiehl, KA, Koenigs, M. Neural correlates of reward and loss sensitivity in psychopathy. *Soc Cogn Affect Neurosci*. 2014; **9**(6): 794–801.

107. Sommer, M, Sodian, B, Döhnel, K, Schwerdtner, J, Meinhardt, J, Hajak, G. In psychopathic patients emotion attribution modulates activity in outcome-related brain areas. *Psychiatry Res*. 2010; **182**(2): 88–95.

108. Dolan, MC, Fullam, RS. Psychopathy and functional magnetic resonance imaging blood oxygenation level-dependent responses to emotional faces in violent patients with schizophrenia. *Biol Psychiatry*. 2009; **66**(6): 570–577.

109. Kumari, V, Das, M, Taylor, PJ, et al. Neural and behavioural responses to threat in men with a history of serious violence and schizophrenia or antisocial personality disorder. *Schizophr Res*. 2009; **110**(1–3): 47–58.

Chapter

9

Political Terrorism and Affective Polarization in "Black" and "Red" Terrorists in Italy During the Years 1968–1988

Matteo Pacini and Icro Maremmani

Introduction

The scientific validity of assessments of violent behavior by means of psychiatric categories has always faced two limitations. On one hand, the controversy about giving political beliefs or activity, or violent behavior in general, a label of mental disturbance was seen as an abuse of psychiatric knowledge. Categorizing politics can lead to justifications of the denigration of certain political ideas as being simply delusional or dangerous, which goes beyond simply being in agreement with the prosecution of perpetrators of violent political acts against the existing regime. The second limitation was that psychiatric evaluations of violent political crimes were mostly performed, case by case, in a forensic environment, which made them unduly dependent on categories of presumed dangerousness and legal responsibility, rather than on a clinical definition of their mental status and history. The forensic classification, in other words, hardly went beyond the distinction between psychotic and nonpsychotic offenders.[1] Psychological theories, mostly based on only a few cases, have gradually increased in number but never led to further, directly related research.[2,3]

Our research group has been investigating the role of bipolar-related states in a variety of events and clinical contexts, such as HIV infection, alcohol abuse by depressed and anxious patients, binge eating, substance abuse, and various kinds of addiction. These studies converged in showing that minor, less-than-manic mood states, including temperamental dispositions (cyclothymic and hyperthymic) are related to a wide range of physiological risk behaviors. For such risks to originate in mood orientation, one does not need to think of a major agitated psychotic mania or mixed state: either a dominant temperament or a protracted hypomania is enough to justify an outcome of engagement in a wide range of activities, whether legal or not, possibly, but not necessarily sociopathic or violent.[4–8] For instance, addiction to alcohol and/or heroin is related to temperamental cyclothymia, rather than axis I dual diagnosis. The move toward sociopathy itself, at least in some cases, may be the result of physiological risk disposition, in a way that does not require the labeling of the resulting behavior (e.g., political violence) as pathological, but makes it interpretable on psychological/clinical grounds.

This paper's aim was to illustrate a series of reports and comments and some data concerning the psychological common ground of political terrorism. To be precise, what we mean by "political terrorism" is an organized and intentional activity that has political aims and is practiced by single individuals or, more often, groups of people who are opposed to a dominant majority, within a certain territory. The choice of terrorism can thus be viewed as a kind of subtle, low-intensity, and scattered war that is focused on politics, rather than a classic struggle for territorial control fought out between armies. It sometimes appears as a civil war, or, more often, implies the clandestine activity of a minority, partly because of the impossibility of sustaining a direct military struggle.

On psychiatric grounds, the focus of our interest is not the political content that is prompted by terrorist movements, nor are we understarting the fact that violent political confrontation is itself a sign of psychiatric orientation. Instead, we are ready to put forward the idea that formal and transpolitical radical choices, either of an illegal lifestyle or of activities involving major risks, can be linked with certain mental states, especially for small groups living in secrecy showing a high level of internal ideological cohesion and a no-return attitude toward commitment to radical choices.

Terrorists usually act in small units, though "lone wolves" exist as well, who may have clear-cut ideological positions, but they remain isolated on the operational plane. Available data about the psycho(patho)logical profile of terrorists are sparse: the few studies that are readily available are those on identified living terrorists (judging by evidence given in the trials of those who personally admitted to having been terrorists), and the statistical data imply a number of documented cases belonging to the same terrorist organization, or at least in the same political area.

Armed political fighting against the system can be distinguished as belonging to one of at least two subtypes, according to Post.[9] On one hand, there are groups fighting for the preservation of their original culture and social environment, in opposition to an enemy that is perceived as "alien," that is, as a hostile force usurping territory, resources, and rights (possibly in a revolutionary mode) or invading from the outside. In addition, there are groups fighting for revolution, aiming at the subversion of what has been considered as normal, or acceptable. This latter kind of terrorism is directed against an inner enemy, which is antagonized but also has shared root features (familial, cultural, ethnic).

As argued by Post, there seems to be a deep difference between those who aim to subvert their own society, the "world of their fathers," and those who, in their view, fight to defend their tradition or retaliate against an attack against the "world of their fathers." The first profile appears to imply a deeper conflict, and a higher level of deviance, among those committed to antitraditional revolutions. Such a statement, as anticipated, does not point to any correspondence between specific contents or a generic judgment of "abnormality" in assessing radicalism, but it suggests that some mental conditions bear a higher likelihood of embracing and engaging in aggressive and outlawed forms of politics, usually on the basis of a radical disagreement with the status quo.

On logical grounds, when terrorists join together as a group, it is quite unlikely that they are in a psychotic state—at least, not all of them at once. It is also unlikely that they feel depressed, or that they are suffering from a severe anxiety disorder, which usually holds people back from making choices, running risks, or engaging in new experiences. Cases of psychotic terrorism take place as isolated attacks, or as very short-lasting participation in group activities. Other categories of mental states show a better fit with a possible long-lasting terrorist activity within the same group, or between similarly oriented groups, which implies a higher level of stability, enduring determination, planning attack campaigns consisting of different actions, and persistent egosyntonia, that is, the situation of someone being convinced that they are fighting to fulfill a right and crucial vow. Mood states of a less-than-manic grade, for instance, would allow an adept to stay within the boundaries of social interaction, military effectiveness, and cautiousness due to a clandestine status, and maintaining a grip on reality, despite an altered set of expectations. The Italian period known familiarly as the "years of lead" displays an interesting viewpoint for the study of terrorist psychology for two main reasons: first, it was a historically defined period (1968–1988); second, the number of ascertained participants in terrorist activities was quite large, especially for the group called the Red Brigades (RBs), the largest European terrorist group known to history. Moreover, a sufficient number of documentaries, interviews, and biographical or true-crime publications are available to allow the possible psychological trajectories of Italian neofascist (right)- and communist (left)-wing extremist groups to be accurately profiled.

Sociology, Existentialism, and Terrorism

The social groundwork that laid the foundations for terrorist choices was identified by Alessandro Orsini[10] as belonging to a socioeconomic process named by him as "progressive deprivation." When this happens, each individual relates him- or herself on one hand to an individual value potential (i.e., what he/she is worth materially in society), and, on the other, to his or her ambitions. Different conditions can develop that place this mechanism of balance under stress. When someone gets poorer, while their ambitions remain the same, we will refer to it as material lessening. When future prospects become uncertain or remain out of sight, people suffer from "ambition deprivation." A further possibility is that someone becomes poorer but is also frustrated about reaching out to achieve any desirable goal, which means perceiving oneself as having become socially marginalized, if not completely excluded. This condition affects a society most deeply when that society undergoes periods of general failure or recession after nurturing the illusion of easy enrichment. On this basis, it becomes more likely that some individuals will react by working out a revolutionary project.

Enrico Fenzi, a former RB militant and university teacher of literature, claims that there was a close relationship between Jean-Paul Sartre's existentialism and the terrorist feelings that were widespread in the 1970s, which he refers to as the "theory of the terrorist group".[11]

Sartre attempts to integrate Marxism (the "class struggle" theory) with his existentialism. He develops a suggestive view, and happens to describe what was actually the psychological experience of those who chose terrorism. You can find an ensemble of objective facts (structural, political . . . put simply, the class struggle), which are enhanced and lead to a critical state, and later to a breaking-point translation into action, because they are coupled to a psychological tension towards personal engagement. Sartre theorizes the psychology of the revolutionary group . . . put more precisely, the subversive group . . . the pure terrorists. On one hand, you have society as it currently exists, with its unacceptable structure (including class divisions), so that everything becomes acceptable to an upside–down view: rebels no longer have any taboos, and, according to the terrorist view, crime in the older form of society is not only acceptable, but, taking into account the premises, looms as the highest conceivable moral position . . . So, it overlaps with what terrorist groups did theorize, in a less elaborate way: friendship is only possible within the group; love is only possible within the group. Being truly human was only possible as long as feelings and relationships were built within the revolutionary project. You could only truly be in love with a comrade; only between those in our group can feelings can be authentic, unlike what happens in the corrupt world outside . . . This search for affective and existential sincerity is only permitted by making a radical choice and maintaining it, whatever the costs may be. Since the most radical of all choices is that of giving a death sentence—death—once this moral obstacle has been overcome, all other choices are automatically cleansed of any element of impurity. [our translation from the Italian]

Beyond this commitment to a fight against society, optimism is another important element. Optimism is not usually attributed to expectation of imminent victory, but rather to an imminent turning point, which will be the beginning of the end for the old world order:

> Without imagining the faith in a reality that would be ready to move after our attempts, this volcano which was about to spit out its lava, certain choices just cannot be understood. At the time, we had that kind

of faith within us. You know, when one thinks about history as an entity which can be influenced and headed where one wants, and you feel you know where it is heading and how you can steer it to the pursued goal . . . it's like a godless religion. We were basically possessed by irrational optimism, because we felt that history was there for us to write it . . . not only that; indeed, we felt we were able to direct it exactly where we would like it to go. [our translation from the Italian]

Another former RB member, Massimo Ghidoni, who once worked as a psychiatrist, compared the full commitment of the terrorist to that of a nun living in seclusion. As he points out, both figures have a view, which works as a flawless belief, but they also feel they are sacrificing their own individual life in favor of the interest of others, aiming at a superior ideal of humanity and society. They both try to act upon reality by the rule of their ideals, instead of remaining isolated in their world of principles. A feeling of compelling love toward humanity is reported by others, too, such as former RB member Valerio Morucci, who played the role of sergeant-at-arms in his unit:

> There was a drive coming from inside . . . a sort of commotion, so strong it could make you break into tears . . . it was not ideology any more at that point . . . It was deeper, and came from an ancient affective core within ourselves.[12]

And again, Roberto Rosso (a former member of the Prima Linea [Front Line] group): "Love—it would become the only and essentially desperate feeling towards the world."[13]

Revolutionary Gnosis

The cognitive array of terrorist groups is structured to convey three basic ideas, which go to make up the revolutionary *gnosis* (i.e., revelation). The first is that a better world is possible but is prevented from coming about by "the system." Mara Cagol, cofounder of the RB, wrote in those terms in a letter to her mother dated in the year 1969: "All the world could live with abundance of goods, but the system does not let that happen." Antagonists to a better world are thought to share the same point of view as those who aim to achieve it. Those antagonists are referred to as incarnating the "counterrevolution," meaning a system of power that is aware of its role, just as it is also aware of the thoughts and aims of revolutionary movements. The second idea is directly dependent on the general "feeling of reality": the terrorist is convinced that victory is potentially imminent, after a final clash. The old world is decadent and about to fall, so revolutionaries should take advantage of this critical stage before the system manages to restore itself in a different form. The third idea, which aims to link up the level of thoughts with that of actions, daringly tries to define the difference between an accomplished revolution and a missed chance in the crucial need to choose the right historical moment. When these ideas get aligned with a manic state, anyone who is fond of revolution, at any time, would be convinced that they possess a clear-cut vision of crucial targets, the right timeframes, and upcoming opportunities. The mood-related urgency to translate theory into practice leads one to set the revolution in motion after the delusion of having run into it by chance. No matter if the underlying spirit is constructive or destructive—this cognitive array takes shape so sharply and rigidly because of its mood-dependent nature. Only a mood-centered vision can combine a sense of the imminence of victory with a sense of positive self-perception, and the expectation that the enemy will turn out to be a fake giant just waiting to be knocked down.

Former RB member Enrico Fenzi gives a fine description of this psychological configuration in his attempt to explain what drove him to leave his family and his job working as a university professor to join the RBs as a clandestine operator:

> Basically . . . the belief was that we were witnessing the downfall of an old world order . . . that a process of deconstruction was going on . . . of society and its values . . . and that we should join in to take part in a turning point, a radical change. We wanted to "be there" while the old society was dying. Joining the Red Brigades implied, at the time, that I would leave my family, my children . . . Why did I do that? . . . because that reality seemed trivial and lessening, if compared with the other perspective, the Armageddon which seemed about to come and subvert everything.

Hypomanic States

It is common to find bipolar traits in the biographies of revolutionary leaders, generals, or people who are either highly constructive or destructive toward the surrounding environment, or simply highly creative.[14] Such a link should at first be conceived as independent from psychiatric categories, and, beyond that, as actively concerned with the physiology of mood states, temperaments, and affective syndromes: it should be understood as an underlying psychobiological model that cannot account for different existential meanings and historical contexts, let alone political views. In other words, bipolar traits can be recognized by their linkage with diametrically opposite political views. As far as deviance is concerned, the concept of pathological deviance is rather intrinsic and implies the impairment of the self as related to one's purposes, whereas no view or idea, no matter how deviant it may be, is intrinsically pathological on psychiatric grounds. Even so, deviant thoughts tend to correspond to a mixed-mania wavelength, which features the urgency to go for some action, or the incapacity to step back instead of striking back, the breadth of goals, and an all-inclusiveness of views.

An individual's existential dimension runs parallel with the historical context, so that the discovery of one's true nature and fate makes one perceive that the whole historical period is experiencing the same change, no matter if some people are still unaware of it, or are even resisting it. This is called the revolutionary *gnosis*, and the *feeling of reality* is the inner mood-dependent state allowing it to reconfigure as a cognitive layout (the *judgment of reality*).

The biographical moment of those who take their chance through political terrorism seems to overlap with a manic-like phase, possibly following a depressive one, so that the new choice may be perceived as "turning a new leaf," a last chance to win one's life back, or the attainment of a level of acute awareness of one's destiny and vocation.

Renato Curcio, a cofounder of the RBs, bridges the social and the existential meanings of revolution (not necessarily of a communist kind) when stating, in an article written in the communist journal *Nuova Resistenza* in 1971, that "the scum of society is the avant-garde of revolution."[10] In addition, this statement recalls the biphasic dynamic of the bipolar cycle (depression-to-mania). In the case of Curcio himself, his biography displays a similar sequence: he was born to an 18-year-old girl, outside marriage, and was fostered by another family during his school years. He would not easily adapt to the rules of a boarding school (he escaped twice, failed twice, and was labeled confrontational and an introvert). At the age of 16, he started his career as a blue-collar worker in Milan, then moved to Genoa by hitchhiking to live there, as a homeless outcast. He eventually found a place to live and a job at the docks, but developed a drinking habit. He describes it as "a hellish period, during which I moved to the brink of a complete mental downfall." This period came to an end when he suddenly made up his mind to leave Genoa and settle down in Trento (feeling "light as a feather"), where he signed up for a university degree course, while moving from one home to another. In the end, he moved back to Milan, where he became committed to political activism, living with other comrades in a community within the urban area. Together with a few others, he decided to live incognito and start a campaign of low-grade terrorist acts. As a sort of rite of passage, he married (in church) his girlfriend and cofounder of the RBs, Mara Cagol, after which they tore up their documents and spent an rather unusual honeymoon planning their future activities.

Homicide and Suicide

By 2008, the cumulative prevalence of suicide in identified terrorists was 13.2 per cent of all causes of death (by comparison, 52.9 per cent died during firefights, using firearms against police forces). It is likely than some unidentified subjects should be included as having committed suicide, as the former left-wing (Lotta Continua) militant Andrea Marcenaro suggested,[15] in speaking about episodes he knew or had learned about. In his explanation, those people fell into a depressive state after taking part in homicides or violent attacks and were haunted by a sense of guilt for having been co-responsible for that pain. Other episodes, though they cannot directly be considered as acts of suicide, can be regarded as parasuicidal. To exemplify, we may quote a report by Enrico Fenzi (the former RB member) about an episode he witnessed during his period in jail: "There have been cases of people who accepted the fact of being killed, just commenting 'all right, I understand you have to kill me, I am to blame, please be quick about it,'" in the kind of context known as a "proletarian trial" (with militants questioning, judging, and sentencing their members or former members who had been accused of betrayal, or of making mistakes, in the same way that would have been used with any "enemy of the people"). To be noticed, the executioners and their victim(s) felt they had to share the same ideological frenzy, somehow sympathizing with each other, going beyond the usual psychology of a death sentence inflicted and suffered, respectively. The victims would approve of their punishments, as if those punishments were due to the only conceivable law—that of revolution. They somehow felt honored to be finished off by their own comrades, which was the only thing they could do in order to "save their soul" and stay consistent with the ideology they had vowed loyalty to. These psychological conditions resemble a (lethal) combination of elated mood states, or a manic and mixed quality, for the executioner(s) and their victim(s), respectively:

> Shortly after his [referring here to an RB member called Giorgio Soldati] arrest ... by the way, I heard they had been roughly beaten up, and so they ended up confessing something, and probably disclosed some names of comrades, charged someone with responsibilities ... He was eventually brought to Cuneo, located in an isolation cell, waiting to be transferred to the regular section with all the others. From his isolation cell, Soldati wrote a letter to his comrades there, and he had it handed over to them, so that when he eventually joined them they would be prepared ... He tried to make excuses, explaining he could not resist the treatment he was given after being arrested ... and so on. And he admitted to naming someone ... He said, "I am sorry, and I am only asking to be judged by my comrades, because they are the only ones I myself give the right to judge me." I am pretty sure that the chiefs read that letter, there's no doubt they did ... It was certainly brought to our cells. Soon after that, Soldati joined us in the regular section ... It was there that ... they called all of us comrades to a meeting ... and he was judged and sentenced to death ... and killed on the spot.

Another RB member, Francesco Berardi, was arrested in Genoa for handing out leaflets of his organization (terrorist propaganda) in the factory where he was a blue-collar worker. He gave testimony about another comrade, Fenzi himself. The two happened to face each other in jail, where Berardi initially looked quite serene, and Fenzi tried to reassure him about the irrelevant weight of his testimony against Berardi (because they added little if any hint of making further accusations), each looking sympathetic toward the other. Nevertheless, Berardi grew more and more upset, and then tried to commit suicide by cutting his wrists. He was rescued, but never recovered, and he refused to ever leave his cell again. He was eventually found dead after hanging himself there.

Suicide, like homicide, is lived through as a form of consistency and loyalty, beyond usual human attitudes about it. Among those who killed their former comrades as betrayers, one can also find examples of this shared mood-related dimension. Roberto Rosso, the former ideological leader of Prima Linea, recalls the reasons that led to the execution of a certain Vaccher, suspected of being a traitor. During the interview reported in the volume *La notte della Repubblica*,[13] he broke into tears and stopped for a while, muttering, "It is awkward to explain . . ." When he recovered and felt ready to continue the interview, the journalist commented, "It must have been even more 'awkward' to do it at the time" [so conveying the sense: that it is "awkward" to explain that now], meaning "How much determination it must have taken to kill a friend just because you felt a suspicion!" What difference stands between then and now? It could be a mood-related one, accounting for the positive value given to deadly actions, which, reconsidered years later, might have become a source of remorse. The decision to inflict death was not painless itself, even at the time, but was subdued to an extreme conception of human relationships, according to which the best relief for pain could be achieved by killing the traitor, in order to preserve the spirit of radical revolution.

Lastly, we would like to recall the case of Roberto Peci, whose brother Patrizio was a leading member of the RBs, but he himself had hardly ever been involved with terrorism, only taking part in minor unarmed actions for a short while. After Patrizio's arrest and confession, the RBs, as a blatant act of revenge, kidnapped Roberto. Nevertheless, Roberto's kidnapping and eventual killing after a death sentence was presented as an act of proletarian justice and explained by the thesis that the two brothers were nothing but infiltrated traitors, who agreed with the police, after fake arrests, to gather information about the RBs and hand them over to official investigators. Roberto's "proletarian trial" was filmed, and he was probably forced to read out a false confession (that he did not feel in any way) that would support the "treason" thesis, so the media would broadcast it as the official truth. He was probably hoping he would be released after consenting to that pantomime, including having him filmed during the reading out of the death sentence—but he was actually killed instead. What counted was that a false confession of treason and commitment to the police was made up, and the life of someone who basically lived outside the world of terrorism was sacrificed in the name of an imminent revolutionary outburst, which would never come, anyway. In the mind of the militants, that killing would act as a spark to light the people's rage against the police and the government, in an optimistically twisted vision of reality, all based on the idea that pushing the right button (in this case, through the media) would be enough to decisively overcome all opposition, in a cascade of revolutionary chaos. Such an idea, the outcome of a mania-like state of mind, now sounds like no more than an optimistic delusion.[16]

"Reds" (Communists) and "Blacks" (Neofascists) Political Terrorists in Italy

Does the general psychological stereotype change according to individual political beliefs? During the period studied by us, it seems possible to indicate a certain difference. Mario Tuti, a fascist militant, once described his extremist drive thus:

> I also regretted having been born too late, and having been unable to take part in World War II, especially in the conclusive phase of defeat, with all the tests of courage and loyalty when others had to prove their worth. At the time . . . I tried to receive some kind of investiture by talking to an old soldier of the Fascist Social Republic, who had not changed his views, and to whom I confessed that a bunch of us were determined to take up arms. I expected moral approval, but he tried to make me think about it again, saying . . . "How do you think you might end up?" I answered that I expected our destiny to be even worse than the destiny they had suffered. He then reminded me that they had experienced only defeat, death, imprisonment, treachery . . . I still remember my words . . . "That's exactly right!"

Curiously, this sounds similar to what the cofounder of the RBs (Alberto Franceschini) reported about his brainstorming encounter with the former communist partisan Giovanbattista Lazagna, who was in arms at the end of World War II, fighting against Nazi and fascist troops in Italy. While expecting some advice from him, or at least some kind of encouragement, he got the following comment, more or less:

> We were fighting with the expectation of a short-term engagement, because the war was reaching its end, and were counting on rather favorable conditions [the allied forces had invaded the country and outnumbered the enemy, who were progressively losing ground]. You, on the other hand, are fancying a struggle that will last for years and years, with no objective point of strength to rely on. It's madness![13]

In both cases, the older comrades discouraged the terrorists-to-be from getting involved in any military conflict. In the first case, however, a pessimistic perspective was a source of fascination for the fascists. In the second, the communists felt unreasonably optimistic about leading a sustainable guerrilla war, and gaining results that were good enough and a degree of consent strong enough to pave the way to a final victory. On the whole, the common ground of political extremism seems to be the mixed-mania stereotype, although starting points may differ: in different historical moments, both major right- and left-wing organizations thought they could take over. Nevertheless, the feeling of the average right-wing extremist was distinguished by a feeling of loneliness, and a lack of mass consent—features that were in contrast with a high level of cultural alignment with the existing world (according to Post, that implied a low level of psychic tension). On the other hand, the Italian left-wing terrorists were aiming to destroy traditional society (according to Post, that implied a high level of psychic tension) but thought they were a living answer to the people's call for freedom. Despite these premises, frustration rose when the course of terrorism found no response in the form of mass approval, let alone insurgence, and the revolutionary spirit was doomed to become more elitist, to shift toward a stronger revolutionary *gnosis*.

Conclusions

In Italy, political terrorism has taken root in the existentialist movement and sociology. Following the "theory of the terrorist group," each terrorist related him- or herself on one hand to an individually assessed potential (i.e., what he/she was worth materially as a member of society) and, on the other, to his or her ambitions. Terrorists considered society as it was at the time, with its unacceptable structure (including class divisions), so that everything became acceptable once an upside–down view was introduced as the new criterion: rebels no longer had any taboos, and, according to the terrorist view, crime in the older form of society was not only acceptable, but, taking into account the premises, loomed as the highest imaginable moral position. The revolutionary *gnosis* was structured to convey three basic ideas: first, that a better world was possible; second, that victory was potentially imminent, after a final clash; and third, that thoughts should lead directly to actions. The biographical stage of those who take their chance through political terrorism seemed to overlap with a manic-like phase, possibly following a depressive one, so that the new choice could be perceived as "turning over a new leaf"—a last chance to win one's life back, or the attainment of a level of acute awareness of one's destiny and vocation. In the personal history of many terrorists, murder and suicide were closely linked. Many terrorists willingly accepted the prospect of being killed by their own comrades, as traitors, even if they had never betrayed anyone. When questioned by the police, they felt guilty, even about having revealed information that was not important and about not having behaved more bravely. If a terrorist is captured, and wants to be killed by his/her own comrades while still in prison, that can certainly be considered a wish to commit suicide. One last consideration is that the general psychological stereotype changed according to individual "red" or "black" beliefs. Remembering the fascist and communist acts during World War II, in both cases, the older party leaders discouraged terrorists-to-be from getting involved in any military conflict. In the first case, however, a pessimistic perspective was a source of fascination for the fascists. In the second, the communists felt unreasonably optimistic about leading a sustainable guerrilla war and gaining a degree of consent strong enough to pave the way to a final victory. On the whole, the common ground of political extremism seems to correspond to the mixed-mania stereotype, although the starting points may differ. In conclusion, beyond a forensic psychiatric evaluation, which goes too far in assessing terrorist acts solely according to categories of presumed dangerousness and legal responsibility, rather than attempting a clinical definition of terrorists' mental status and history, a relationship between terrorism and affective polarization does exist.

Disclosures

Matteo Pacini does not have anything to disclose. Icro Maremmani declares personal fees from Indivior, Molten, Gilead, Mundipharma, and from MSD, with no relation with the present paper.

References

1. Kalian, M, Zabow, A, Witztum, E. Political assassins—the psychiatric perspective and beyond. *Med Law*. 2003; **22**(1): 113–130.

2. Miller, L. The terrorist mind, II: typologies, psychopathologies, and practical guidelines for investigation. *Int J Offender Ther Comp Criminol*. 2006; **50**(3): 255–268.

3. Miller, L. The terrorist mind, I: a psychological and political analysis. *Int J Offender Ther Comp Criminol*. 2006; **50**(2): 121–138.

4. Bacciardi, S, Maremmani, I, Rovai, L, et al. Drug (heroin) addiction, bipolar spectrum and impulse control disorders. *Heroin Addict Relat Clin Probl*. 2013; **15**(2): 29–36.

5. Maremmani, I, Pacini, M, Perugi, G, Deltito, J, Akiskal, H. Cocaine abuse and the bipolar spectrum in 1090 heroin addicts: clinical observations and a proposed pathophysiologic model. *J Affect Disord*. 2008; **106**(1–2): 55–61.

6. Maremmani, I, Lazzeri, A, Pacini, M, Lovrecic, M, Placidi, GF, Perugi, G. Diagnostic and symptomatological features in chronic psychotic patients according to cannabis use status. *J Psychoactive Drugs*. 2004; **36**(2): 235–241.

7. Maremmani, AG, Rugani, F, Bacciardi, S, et al. Does dual diagnosis affect violence and moderate/superficial self-harm in heroin addiction at treatment entry? *J Addict Med.* 2014; **8**(2): 116–122.

8. Rugani, F, Bacciardi, S, Rovai, L, et al. Symptomatological features of patients with and without ecstasy use during their first psychotic episode. *Int J Environ Res Public Health.* 2012; **9**(7): 2283–2292.

9. Post, JM. Terrorist on trial: the context of political crime. *J Am Acad Psychiatry Law.* 2000; **28**(2): 171–178.

10. Orsini, A. *Anatomia delle Brigate Rosse: Le Radici Ideologiche del Terrorismo Rivoluzionario Storia e Società* [in Italian]. Soveria Mannelli, Italy: Rubettino; 2010.

11. Fenzi, E. *Armi e Bagagli: Un Diario dalle Brigate Rosse* [in Italian]. Milano: Costa & Nola; 1987.

12. Morucci, V. *La Peggio Gioventù: Una Vita nella Lotta Armata* [in Italian]. Milano: Rizzoli; 2004.

13. Zavoli, S. *La Notte della Repubblica* [in Italian]. Milano: Mondadori; 1995.

14. Akiskal, KK, Akiskal, HS. The theoretical underpinnings of affective temperaments: implications for evolutionary foundations of bipolar disorder and human nature. *J Affect Disord.* 2005; **85**(1–2): 231–239.

15. Trotta, R. La colonna. In: *La Grande Storia* [in Italian]. Roma: Radiotelevisione Italiana; 2000.

16. Perotti, LM. director. *L'infame e Suo Fratello* [film, in Italian]. Tamarama, New South Wales, Australia: Stamen Films; 2008. www.Lastoriasiamonoi.Rai.It/Puntate/Linfame-E-Suo-Fratello/821/Default.Aspx; 2008. Accessed July 5, 2017.

Chapter 10

Conditions of Life and Death of Psychiatric Patients in France During World War II: Euthanasia or Collateral Casualties?

Patrick Lemoine and Stephen M. Stahl

Introduction

Euthanasia of tens of thousands of German psychiatric patients (as many as 200,000) by the Nazis in the T4 and other related programs is now well known.[1,2] It is also widely known that more than 48,000 French psychiatric patients died of hunger, exposure, indifference, and oblivion during the early 1940s while France was under Nazi control and while gassing, cremation, and starvation of children with disabilities was occurring inside Germany.[3,4] In 1936, before the start of World War II and the Nazi occupation of France, Alexis Carrel, an American Nobel Prize Winner of French descent, published *Man: The Unknown*,[5] in which the horror of psychiatric eugenics—with mass involuntary sterilization of psychiatric patients—was made plain for all to see. He would go on to become one of the main intellectual forces in the Vichy government. However, at the same time his book was published, and when the world had already halted involuntary sterilization of psychiatric patients, Nazi psychiatrists moved from sterilization to euthanasia of disabled patients, and tens of thousands made their way to gas chambers or were killed by involuntary starvation or barbiturate overdose as the notorious T4 operation and its successors got under way in Germany.[1,2]

Was psychiatric euthanasia by starvation occurring simultaneously in Nazi-occupied France? The figures speak for themselves: 48,588 additional deaths in psychiatric hospitals occurred between 1940 and 1944. In order to have a better understanding of these events, it is helpful to look into one of these hospitals, the Hôpital du Vinatier, a psychiatric facility in Lyon, the country's second largest city, in the center of France, and where the principal author of the present article (PL) spent many years as a practicing psychiatrist. The present manuscript will refer to original materials referenced and reproduced in an account written by the principal author based on the real history of people who lived at Hôpital du Vinatier in Lyon-Bron during World War II.[6] Dr. Lemoine has also researched the hospital files at Vinatier and interviewed survivors involved with the hospital during that era. In addition, the book contains several facsimiles and documents (many in French and others in English or German), including: an introduction to Rochaix's report, extracts of Vinatier's report to de Gaulle, a letter from a representative of the general council, and more. The reader is referred to the book[6] for more detailed references and documents. What follows herein is a summary of the story of Vinatier from the authors' perspectives, published now in English, so that a shorter version can reach more readers.

The Context

In 1938, as the rumors of war began to take shape, the board of the Hôpital du Vinatier decided to purchase 300 gasmasks for some of its personnel (i.e., employees and working patients). The latter were considered "good patients" by hospital personnel, because without them the hospital could not function. These "good patients" were in charge of day-to-day chores and supplies: cleaning, washing up, farming, laundry, and domestic service for the directors and doctors. How about the other 2,900 patients in the event of a gas attack? Hospital policy was as follows: "They had to take refuge in the ditches,"[6] a measure whose effectiveness against poison gas was highly questionable, since combat gas was designed to accumulate in trenches. This was a year before the war, but not one voice was raised in protest against the policy. All this seems to indicate a willingness to sacrifice psychiatric patients for the good of others.

According to accounts of the time, money did not run short at the hospital.[6] Far from it. That same year, on March 28, 1938, Hôpital du Vinatier purchased a bas relief by Jean Chorel, a well-known Lyonnais sculptor. It was an imitation stone proof of his "Les Boeufs" [The Oxen], a gold medalist at the Salon de Paris of 1934. Instead of purchasing this relief, many doctors had requested that the money be allocated for purchase of an X-ray device on account of the high incidence of pulmonary tuberculosis. Their request was met with a staunch refusal.

To set the background and environment in which Vinatier functioned at that time, in 1938, Professor Anthelme Rochaix, who held the chair of Hygienics at the University of Lyon and was also the brother of a psychiatrist and the head doctor at Hôpital du Vinatier, was commissioned by the authorities to write a report entitled "A Report on the Struggle Against Pathological Heredity." The report read as follows: "Life expectancy amongst human beings is getting considerably longer. In consequence of which there is an increase in the number of degenerate and defective beings, i.e., the dregs of the earth, who, as a result of the suppression of the law of natural selection, contribute to the degeneracy of the race and become a heavy burden for the community."[6] The remainder of the report is rather moderate and merely raises queries.

Times of Crisis

According to the official version of events, all these wasted lives (i.e., 2,000 additional deaths at Hôpital du Vinatier alone), hinge on a sheer "omission" by the Vichy government—namely, an inability to provide enough food for all. The dietary requirements (1,427 calories, as stated on official ration cards), which the entire French population was supposed to be provided, were not enough. Only the ingenuity of the civilian population helped them to survive: the development of a black market, small plots of land rented out for gardening, relatives in the countryside, etc. People were hungry, but they did not starve since the comparative death rate among the civilian population was no higher than 1 per cent during the war.

A map was made of all hospitals, convalescent homes, sanatoriums, and other sanitary institutions, though it left out psychiatric hospitals and prisons. Conventional prisons, it seems, were able to set up an efficient black market because the mortality rate among prisoners remained stable. Unfortunately, insane patients had neither the financial nor psychological means. They fell like flies. Between December 1939 and March 1946, 47.7 per cent of psychiatric patients at the hospital in Isère starved to death.[4] In 1942 alone, 41.98 per cent of patients at the Hôpital du Vinatier were carried away amid the turmoil.[6] In terms of percentages, it is perhaps the worst massacre in the history of France.

In 1944, near the end of the war, because of the great number of deaths among psychiatric patients, there was a lot of free space at the Hôpital du Vinatier, and so a neurology unit was transferred there. As these neurology patients were not mentally ill, the directorship found it only too natural to grant them larger rations than those given to other inpatients. Once again, no one dared utter a word of protest. Only the pharmacist and a few doctors bravely tried to fight this injustice, but their means were very limited. Once again, this indicated the willingness of hospital officials to sacrifice the mentally ill for more "meritorious" patients.

There had been no actual proof of official intention in terms of eugenics, no documents, no "smoking gun."[6] The historian Isabelle von Bueitzingslowen was granted permission by Hôpital Vinatier to conduct a research project that would enable denial of any intentionality involved in the "psychiatric hecatomb," to determine that there was no policy of purposely sacrificing the mentally ill for the good of the many. She found exactly the same number of casualties as had been previously widely reported (2,000 additional deaths) but argued that, since she could find no official documents condoning or ordering a policy of purposely starving psychiatric patients so that the food could be used by others, these deaths and the starvation that occurred could not have been intentional.[7] For her, the absence of evidence was evidence of absence. Recall, however, that Hitler himself strictly forbade any issuance of written documents related to the T4 project of euthanasia in Germany, and instead "medicalized" it, while having psychiatrists administer the means of death under the guise of treatment.[1,2]

Thus, the most widespread explanation put forward for the deaths at Vinatier during this era was a lack of food. But that is a difficult conclusion to support because at Vinatier there was a hospital farm, in fact the finest in the region (about 800,000 square meters, or about 200 acres, plus 80 cows and 600 pigs), which, if well managed, would have produced enough food to avoid starvation among Vinatier patients. Before the war, in fact, the farm provided a third of the food supplies for the patients as well as additional rations given as bonuses for nurses. Though initially in a state of collapse at the beginning of World War II, the farm nevertheless all the while continued to sell foodstuffs to the outside world. The psychiatric patients at Vinatier were literally starving in the midst of plenty. Was this an accident, thousands of "collateral casualties," or was it due to a policy of psychiatric euthanasia by starvation, sacrificing the mentally ill so that the food could go to others? One had to wait until 1942 for a change of management at Vinatier, when at last a competent person was appointed, and the following year, in 1943, food production picked up considerably. The mortality rate at Vinatier also began to drop at the same time.

To a great extent, the problem of patients starving at Vinatier was completely denied at the time. According to Dr. P. Scherrer, following his experience at Auxerre, "the nurses who lived through this period try and forget by denying these impossible deaths."[8] The majority of nurses who worked at Vinatier during this era and were interviewed by our principal author remain persuaded that it was all due to a "strange epidemic."

The Post-War Years

In 1946, probably spurred on by General de Gaulle, the government requested a report from all hospitals "concerning the years of crisis." Hôpital du Vinatier's report was issued in 1947. All aspects were mentioned: the admissions, the discharges, the deaths. "The hospital has constantly applied rationing according to the plan by the Office of General Supplies."[6] The message could not have been clearer. The response from the Regional Council was no less explicit and needs no comment: "All the departmental counselors have been given this extremely interesting report. Your local commission insisted on praising the board of Hôpital du Vinatier for having succeeded in submitting such a comprehensive document on the functioning of your hospital."[6] Officially, starvation of psychiatric patients (strictly applying rationing of calories to psychiatric patients) was thus condoned. No others were so rationed. Did this imply that the lives of psychiatric patients were less worthwhile and deserved rationing and starvation while others did not?

A Parallel Between France and Germany?

On September 1, 1939, Hitler gave orders to start operation T4.[2] Psychiatric experts in Germany analyzed the medical files of patients in order to sort out the curable from the incurably ill. Within only a few months, many tens of thousands of patients, mostly children, deemed to be incurable, were exterminated in gas chambers built inside the psychiatric hospitals.[1,2] The families were then informed that their relatives had been carried off by an infectious disease and that their corpses had been cremated in order to avoid any risk of epidemic. However, the secret program was soon laid wide open. The German population began to protest against the active gassing of patients. Petitions flooded in, sometimes even from advocates of Nazism who could not bear their relatives being exterminated. So the Nazis turned to "wild euthanasia," which encouraged continued death to psychiatric patients but no longer centrally administered, so that the gassing and cremation stopped, and a program of starvation was instituted.[1,2] Obviously, in retrospect, the Nazis had bigger plans for how to use gassing and cremation in Poland and other concentration camps for the "Final Solution." Allowing psychiatric patients to starve to death was "more natural" and therefore more likely to be accepted and understood by the general population, and this would disguise the fact that this was really a form of euthanasia. In the final analysis, more than 200,000 mentally ill Germans died in this manner during the war.[1,2] An order was also given not to keep any written records of the program.

The Stands Taken by the Allies

In the newspaper *La Raison* in 1952,[9] there was an eyewitness account of a 1947 conversation at the Nuremberg trials with a Dr. Pfanmueller, a psychiatrist and the director of an asylum.[1,2] One witness, a Mr. Lehner, quoted Pfanmueller thus:

> To me, of course, as a national socialist, these creatures represent but a burden on the healthy body of our country. We do not get rid of them by means of poison or injections, as that would provide the foreign press with hate propaganda. No. Our method is a lot simpler and far more natural, as you may see.

After speaking these words, Pfanmueller dragged a child out of bed. As he displayed the infant like one might a dead hare, he said that this would still take another two or three days:

> I can still vividly remember this fat man, grinning sardonically, holding in his large hands this small skeleton breathing amongst other starving children. Dr. Pfanmueller stated that they would not be abruptly deprived of food, though the rations would be gradually reduced.

The Nuremberg prosecutor examining Pfanmueller on the witness stand made some calculations: "Thus, between November 12th and December 1st, 1940, you have sent more than two thousand questionnaires. By working ten hours a day, you would have been able to do a hundred and one a day, spending five minutes on each."[6,9] This only goes to prove that such assessments were more than cursory, to say the least.[1,2]

On November 8, 1949, *Die Neue Zeitung* published an article concerning Pfanmueller, whom the Court of Assizes of Munich had just sentenced to six years imprisonment.[1,2,6,9] The court judged that "the extermination of mentally ill patients was not murder but manslaughter that may have been involuntary."[1,2] So Pfanmueller was spared the death penalty and given a relatively light sentence.

It seems clear here that, on the one hand, under certain ideological conditions during a crisis situation of World War II, psychiatrists may have knowingly allowed patients to starve to death or even killed them with their own hands.[1,2] On the other hand, after the war was over in 1946–1947, Western authorities considered there to be a difference between the life of someone who was mentally ill and that of a mentally healthy or so-called "normal person." Purposely causing the death of a mentally ill person was not murder, but involuntary manslaughter?

The Question of Eugenics

One question appears to be essential: Were the starvation deaths of psychiatric patients a case of euthanasia in France in general, or at Vinatier in particular? One must not lose sight of the fact that everything regarding the extermination of mentally ill persons had to be kept strictly secret, which has made historical research most difficult. The Nazis strongly insisted on this, as clearly indicated in several documents printed in the review *La Raison*.[1,2,6] Orders in this Nazi operation were mostly given orally. Besides, it was reported in the same issue[6] that "Late in 1942, the directors of psychiatric asylums in Germany were given orders to slowly starve these useless eaters to death. This method was found to be excellent, as death seemed natural."

The parallel with the situation in France is indeed disturbing. As of yet, there is no definitive proof that when Hitler became aware of the public reaction regarding gas chamber exterminations he then applied the same policy of starvation of mentally ill patients in occupied countries as well. Nevertheless, it is difficult to believe that the Nazis—who applied racist and eugenic policies with regard to a number of minority groups in France—would have made an exception for the mentally ill. Yet, one could suggest the possibility that the policy applied in France resulted using the same methods: no written orders and only oral instructions to a certain number of directors of psychiatric asylums who were considered reliable. For instance, the prefect in Lyon, a Mr. Angeli, faithful to Pierre Laval (a prominent minister in Marshall Petain's Vichy government), was a Nazi henchman and notorious collaborator who was later imprisoned and sentenced to death during the Liberation.

The director of Hôpital du Vinatier came from the staff of the Prefecture of Lyon, who had been appointed before the war. The attitude of this director was ambiguous: the man in charge of the farm was a prisoner of war, who appointed someone else who was incompetent and who did not seem to worry about the drop-off in agricultural production. He lowered the wages of patient workers without explanation, despite the hospital's enormous financial assets. He also did not support the black market and stuck strictly to the official ration policies.

According to Odier,[4] Vichy's project, if there has ever been any at all, did not aim at systematic extermination. So then at this stage, if we are not speaking of intentional extermination, could we not at least speak of negligence? Those who had degraded lives—such as they were believed to be—were gradually led to voluntary euthanasia. In fact, this project may well have intended to rid psychiatric hospitals of the incurably ill in order to free up resources for those individuals that the institution still had great hopes to heal. When it came down to diseases detected at an early stage in children, it was deemed necessary to separate the curable from the incurably ill, and the doctors' help was requested by the General Supplies Office. Fifty years removed from the event, it is nonetheless difficult to say if that selection indeed took place. In case it did happen, one can understand why the doctors have kept silent about it.

This assertion is supported by an official social services document from the Department of Health, 22nd Sanitary District, General Director's Office, at the directorship of Saint-Robert's Psychiatric Asylum in Grenoble:

> As regards additional milk or low-fat cheese, ask your doctors to name the beneficiaries according to a distinct order as follows: treatable patients, i.e., those who will, after receiving adequate treatment and a short stay at your hospital, be able to regain their freedom and take up their former places in society as well as their previous occupations. These are the ones who ought to take food again. However, for those who will soon be terminally ill, and of whom I have seen a great number during my last visit, it is not possible to make a dent in the General Food Supplies, as they are in difficulties at the present time.[6]

Had there really been a deliberate policy of active euthanasia of psychiatric patients in France? Such authors as Dr. Lucien Bonnafé (1912–2003)[6] do not hesitate to take that plunge:

> Considerable overcrowding in psychiatric hospitals was already a problem before the war. The fascist policy of "assistance" to the mentally ill as applied by the occupied forces and the Vichy government was a way to come up with a drastic solution: 40,000 mental patients died of hunger and exposure during the war.

Professor Rochaix's inconclusive report (mentioned and referenced[6] above), which was requested and backed by the authorities at that time, displays the eugenic atmosphere that was prevalent before the war. The refusal to purchase gasmasks for unemployed patients, accompanied by the recommendation that able-bodied patients be sent to the wide ditches, only confirms an intention to exterminate. At the very least, it conveyed a certain degree of cynicism tinged with heedlessness. Many additional clues are also provided about the eugenic climate of the time, such as the absence of official protest when the supervisory board decided to allot extra food supplies to the transferred patients under the pretext that they were entitled to it since they were not psychiatric patients. In addition, there were unjustified budget cuts concerning "recreational activities for the patients."

In addition, it is interesting to make a comparison with what took place at other similar hospitals that were able to avoid the increased number of deaths. In Saint-Jean de Dieu (a private psychiatric hospital in Lyon, 3 km from Vinatier), at the hospital Sainte Marie du Puy in Rodez, and at the psychiatric hospital in Saint Alban, a similar slaughter was avoided by the determination and imagination of those in charge. They were able to inflict punishment for food theft, cultivate every available plot of land, and encourage the black market. At Vinatier, they let the farm fall into ruin, and only the staff took advantage of cultivated plots. Food thefts by the staff seemed to have been significant, but they were not subject to strong punishment. It was not until 1942 that a new director was nominated and a competent farm manager appointed. Within a year, the mortality curve was inverted dramatically. Also in 1942, a new recommendation by the Department of State for Health authorized psychiatric hospitals to provide supplementary food in psychiatric hospitals.

During the Liberation, there was no official reaction to what happened to these psychiatric patients. No inquiry was called for by the new government, though the truth was immediately disclosed. On September 26, 1945, a Mr. Billoux, Minister of Health, stated the following in a speech at the Vélodrome d'Hiver: "The number of mentally ill persons has decreased substantially since 1939. One must take into account the fact that many of those hospitalized at psychiatric asylums have literally starved to death."[6] One Dr. Dugoujon,[6] a departmental counselor and a friend of Jean Moulin (a greatly respected hero and martyr of the Resistance), congratulated Vinatier's directorship on their "extremely interesting report." Quite recently, in fact, he told the principal author that, at the time of the Liberation, "I had not read this report, as we had other fish to fry!"

Even in times of peace, anti-psychiatric racism is an underlying problem that lurks in the shadows. This can be seen, for instance, by the sterilization of sick people, carried out without personal consent in the early twentieth century in France, Sweden, and the United States. It is also attested to by the exclusion of coverage of mental illness in certain insurance contracts today.

But in times of crisis, this is even more brutally expressed, as can be seen based on the evidence of psychiatric gulags and recent events that occurred in Romania.

Psychiatric eugenics can be found in a more or less assertive, conscious manner, in every man, because "aliéné" (an insane person) means, etymologically, "the other" (from Latin "alienus"). This represents the unbearable madness that we all fear lies within each of us. A lunatic is also the weakest one among us, making him the ideal scapegoat. The histories of insanity and of civilizations are one and the same, because the manner in which society treats the insane reflects its representations of otherness. According to R. Girard from Stanford University, when a community goes through a crisis and its identity structures are put in jeopardy, the need arises for a sacrificial victim whose appointment will be based first and foremost on the notion of difference.[6] Even if they are compelled by widespread tensions beyond their grasp, which they are generally not conscious of, decision makers do not usually make generous gifts to the most different of citizens—the mentally ill. The "Other," "l'Aliéné," is the ideal victim—discreet and silent.

The concept of "the other" is certainly not a new one. World War II was not the first time it was prominent, nor will it be the last. By pushing a group of people into the category of the "other," it is much easier to dehumanize them and thereby justify any actions, no matter how vile, committed against them. This method of "othering" has been used successfully by propaganda campaigns throughout history to justify racism, sexism, war, and many of the most gruesome acts of violence. It can be seen in action constantly throughout the globe: in long-running civil wars, in arguments over whether or not to accept refugees during times of crisis, or during political campaigns when both sides attack each another. Everyone wants someone to blame for things not being as they should be. Having a common enemy to hate can provide a strong bond among allies.

One of the most complicated examples of this phenomenon today would be terrorism and the work of the so-called Islamic State. ISIL has been quite masterful at employing propaganda campaigns through social media and viral videos. Following the lead of many who came before them, they first created a group that would serve as "the other." In their case, it is not only the "West" but also those in the Middle East who do not share their values: Christians, Jews, Yazidis, and the "wrong kind of Muslims" (i.e., Shiites). Members of these groups are lumped together as having the wrong values, and are then dehumanized, demonized, and made to be seen as the reason for all the problems that exist in the world. Any violent acts committed against the so-called "others" can then be not only justified but perceived as more than warranted—as righteous.

One of the most important lessons, then, that the T4 program and its effects in Germany, in France, and globally teaches us is how crucial it is to admit to our mistakes instead of denying them or trying to hide from them —how vital it is to acknowledge an ugly truth and admit to ourselves that humankind has an enormous propensity for weakness and brutality. In this way, we can hopefully remember that each of us is, in fact, an "other."

Disclosures

Patrick Lemoine does not have anything to disclose.

Stephen M. Stahl, M.D., Ph.D., is an adjunct professor of psychiatry at the University of California–San Diego, an honorary visiting senior fellow at the University of Cambridge (UK), and director of psychopharmacology for the California Department of State Hospitals. Over the past 36 months, he has served as a consultant to Acadia, Alkermes, Allergan, Arbor Pharmaceuticals, AstraZeneca, Avanir, Axovant, Axsome, Biogen, Biomarin, Biopharma, Celgene, DepoMed, Dey, EnVivo, Fanapt, Forest, Forum, Genomind, Innovative Science Solutions, Intra-Cellular Therapies, Jazz, Lilly, Lundbeck, Merck, Novartis, Noveida, Orexigen, Otsuka, PamLabs, Perrigo, Pierre Fabre, Reviva, Servier, Shire, Sprout, Sunovion, Taisho, Takeda, Teva, Tonix, Trius, and Vanda. He is a board member of RCT Logic and Genomind. He has served on the speakers bureaus for Astra Zeneca, Dey Pharma, EnVivo, Eli Lilly, Forum, Genentech, Janssen, Lundbeck, Merck, Otsuka, PamLabs, Pfizer Israel, Servier, Sunovion, and Takeda. He has received research and/or grant support from Acadia, Alkermes, AssureX, Astra Zeneca, Arbor Pharmaceuticals, Avanir, Axovant, Biogen, Braeburn Pharmaceuticals, BristolMyer Squibb, Celgene, CeNeRx, Cephalon, Dey, Eli Lilly, EnVivo, Forest, Forum, GenOmind, GlaxoSmithKline, Intra-Cellular Therapies, ISSWSH, Janssen, JayMac, Jazz, Lundbeck, Merck, Mylan, Neurocrine, Neuronetics, Novartis, Otsuka, PamLabs, Pfizer, Reviva, Roche, Sepracor, Servier, Shire, Sprout, Sunovion, TMS NeuroHealth Centers, Takeda, Teva, Tonix, Vanda, Valeant, and Wyeth. He also holds stock options from Genomind and Adamas.

References

1. Burleigh, M. *Death and Deliverance: Euthanasia in Germany 1900–1945*. Cambridge: Cambridge University Press; 1994.

2. Friedlander, H. *The Origins of Nazi Genocide: From Euthanasia to the Final Solution*. Chapel Hill, NC: University of North Carolina Press; 1995.

3. Lafont, M. L'extermination douce [The gentle extermination] [in French]. Doctoral dissertation. Lyon: Université de Médecine Claude Bernard; 1981.

4. Odier, S. Conditions matérielles d'internement dans un hôpital psychiatrique (1930–1960) [Material conditions of detention in a psychiatric hospital (1930–1960)] [in French]. Master's thesis. Lyon: Université de Lyon; 1992.

5. Carrel, A. *Man: The Unknown*. Garden City, NY: Halcyon House; 1938.

6. Lemoine, P. *Droit d'asiles [Right of Asylum]* [in French]. Paris: Odile Jacob Press; 1998.

7. Von Bueitzingslowen, I. *L'Hécatombe des fous: La Famine dans les Hôpitaux Psychiatriques français sous l'Occupation* [*Sacrifice of the Insane: Famine in the French Psychiatric Hospitals under the Occupation*] [*in French*]. Paris: Aubier; 2007.

8. Scherrer, P. *L'hôpital libéré [The Liberated Hospital]* [in French]. Paris: Éditions Atelier Alpha-Bleue; 1989.

9. Anonymous. *La Raison* [Paris newspaper]. 1952; **35**: 37, 38.

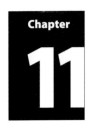

Chapter

11

Neuropsychiatric Characteristics of Antiterrorist Operation Combatants in the Donbass (Ukraine)

Konstantin N. Loganovsky, Natalia A. Zdanevich, Marina V. Gresko, Donatella Marazziti, and Tatiana K. Loganovskaja

Introduction

War will always have physical and psychological effects on all of the people involved—soldiers and civilians, including the contingents of refugees, migrants, prisoners, hostages, and residents from the involved territories. War can lead to radical changes in every aspect of life, even to the point where time is henceforth demarcated as "before the war" and "after the war."

Considerations about the undoubted effects of war on mental health depend significantly on the social and political structures of the affected populations. According to *The Experience of Soviet Medicine in the Great Patriotic War of 1941–1945*,[1] the "high consciousness and true patriotism of the Soviet soldier caused a significant overall reduction of neuroses in the army and an extremely favorable clinical course of neurotic diseases." Obviously, this is pure Soviet propaganda. Indeed, according to the evidence-based data, mental health disorders and associated psychosomatic disorders among participants in armed conflict causes huge medical and social burdens everywhere.[2,3] Not surprisingly, the prevalence of posttraumatic stress disorder (PTSD) is 0.3–6.1 per cent in the general population, but its rate in individuals who have faced war is 15.4 per cent.[2,4]

Mental health is defined as a state of well-being in which an individual realizes his or her own potential, can cope with the normal stresses of life, can work productively and fruitfully, and is able to make a contribution to her or his community.[5] In this sense, mental health is the basis of well-being and effective functioning for the individual and their society. Mental health depends upon and simultaneously significantly affects physical health and socioeconomic circumstances.

The psycho/pathological effects of emergency situations have been described since the occurrence of the American Civil War (1861–1865) under the form of the psychological and psychosomatic consequences that have been widely confirmed after subsequent conflicts. Other dramatic emergencies—like nuclear power plant disasters and earthquakes—have been reported to provoke depression, anxiety, PTSD, substance-related and addictive disorders, and a variety of medically unexplained symptoms.[6–8]

Since the Chernobyl disaster, another traumatic crisis, the war in the Donets Basin (the Donbass) has occurred in Ukraine, and it has had a massive impact on Ukrainian society. Before this war, 3.8 million people lived in the occupied territories of the Donbass. That number is now close to 2 million, as 1.8 millions have escaped to the western parts of the country and become internally displaced persons (refugees and migrants). Around 150,000 combatants have participated in antiterrorism operations (ATO) there. The conflict has resulted in a dramatic and long-term deterioration of the mental and physical health of all its participants.[9–18] Resolution and possible prevention of such consequences will most probably require institution of an integrated biopsychosocial approach.

The goal of the present study was to explore the neuropsychiatric characteristics of the ATO combatants in the Donbass and to propose therapeutic strategies for managing their mental healthcare.

Subjects and Methods

In the period January 2015–May 2016, a random sample (the study group) of 54 ATO combatants (53 men and 1 woman, mean age±SD = 30.8±8.2 years) underwent inpatient psychological, neurological, and psychiatric assessment and given care at the Department of Radiation Psychoneurology of the National Research Center for Radiation Medicine of the National Academy of Medical Sciences (NRCRM) in Kyiv. The distribution of soldiers by military unit is depicted in Figure 11.1. It should be emphasized that almost all surveyed ATO participants were under the constant patronage of volunteers from nongovernmental organizations (NGOs). All the examined ATO combatants took

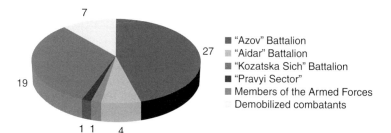

Figure 11.1. Distribution of ATO combatants (n = 54) by military units (the Azo, Aidar, Kozatska, and Pravyi groups were volunteers).

part in continuous active fighting (combat exposure range = one month to two years; mean = one year). ATO combatants from the Military Forces of Ukraine were reservists who had served before in the army (USSR or Ukraine). Volunteers (the "Aidar," "Azov," "Kozatska," and "Pravyi" groups) belonged to the Euromaidan movement and were former civilians.

In order to compare the mental state of the ATO combatants with that of other subjects exposed to emergencies, the following groups were employed for comparisons:

- Group A: individuals exposed in utero and at 0–1 years of age at the time of the Chernobyl disaster (April 26, 1986) and a control group of unexposed persons of the same age (n = 189 and 139, respectively; mean age±SD = 25.5±5.8 years).
- Group B: cleanup workers from the Chernobyl accident (liquidators, n = 81, mean age±SD = 55.5±6.6 years) suffering from PTSD and comorbid chronic cerebrovascular pathology.
- Group C: subjects evacuated from the Chernobyl exclusion zone (n = 76, mean age±SD = 50.7±8.0 years) suffering from PTSD and comorbid chronic cerebrovascular pathologies.
- Group D: veterans of the Afghan War (n = 28, mean age±SD = 47.2±6.3 years) with PTSD following a closed head injury.

Diagnosis of psychiatric, behavioral, and central nervous system (CNS) disorders was carried out according to the criteria of the International Statistical Classification of Diseases and Related Health Problems, 10th revision (ICD–10).[19]

The Mini-Mental State Examination (MMSE) was employed to screen for cognitive impairment.[20] This scale is the one most often used in modern epidemiological and clinical studies to assess overall mental status and includes several subtests that allow for a quick and effective evaluation of orientation in time, place, and state; short- and long-term memory; language function; gnosis; and praxis (i.e., the basic cognitive functions). Scoring levels for the MMSE were categorized as follows: 28–30 = without cognitive deficit (almost healthy); 24–27 = mild cognitive impairment; ≤23 = dementia.

The following scales were utilized for qualitative and quantitative evaluation of psychopathological symptoms, personality disorders, and psychiatric disorders: (1) the General Health Questionnaire (GHQ–28), which measures somatoform symptoms, anxiety/insomnia, social dysfunction, and severe depression;[21,22] (2) the Zung Self-Rating Depression Scale (SRDS) for depression;[23] and (3) PTSD was assessed with the Impact of Events Scale (IES), the Irritability, Depression, Anxiety (IDA) Scale, and the Mississippi Scale for Combat-Related PTSD (M–PTSD). These self-rating scales evaluate the characteristic symptoms of PTSD and are generally used to study psychological distress.[24–26]

Two personality profile analyses—one before ATO participation (retrospectively) and one at the time of the survey—were carried out to investigate possible individual personality changes following combat operations. The questionnaires used for this purpose were the Questionnaire for the Determination of Accentuated Personalities[27] and the Eysenck Personality Questionnaire.[28,29]

The functional state of the brain was evaluated using quantitative electroencephalography (qEEG), based on topographic mapping with a 16-channel analyzer DX-4000 (Kyiv, Ukraine). Spectral power and visual EEG analyses were also performed. In order to study cerebral hemodynamics, ultrasound duplex scanning of the extracranial parts of the brachiocephalic vessels with cerebral insonation (Willis' circle) on the front and rear occipital temporal ultrasound window was carried out with the SonoAce 9900 and 8000 apparatus (Medison, Seoul, Korea).

Excel 2010 spreadsheets were employed to structure our database. Statistical analysis was performed by parametric and nonparametric analyses with Statistica software (v. 10.0, StatSoft, San Francisco, California).

Results

A comparison of the ages of the study groups showed that the age of ATO combatants ($M \pm SD$ = 30.8±8.2 years) was higher than that of group A (25.5±5.8 years), but lower than that of groups B (55.5±6.6 years), C (50.7±8.0 years), and D (47.2±6.3 years).

The most frequent complaints of ATO combatants were as follows: permanent diffuse headache, dizziness, tinnitus, hearing loss, back pain along the spine, blurred vision, heart discomfort, poor sleep involving dreams with military themes, anxiety, depressive mood, emotional tension, irritability, confusion, and persistent memories of combat situations.

On neuropsychiatric examination, they were found to have clear consciousness, productive contacts, and full orientation toward time, space, and personality. Their insight was mainly preserved, and their thought process was logical. Their main complaints were emotional lability, anxiety, tension, dyssomnia, psychopathological phenomena, "flashbacks" (retrospection, "looking back," "reverse shot"), increased irritability, and physiological reactivity. Their language (speech) skills were not impaired.

The most common neurological symptoms were dizziness, dyscoordination, and ataxia, suggestive of cerebellum and brain stem impairment, while the pyramidal and extrapyramidal systems and sensitivity were less involved. In contrast, a marked paravertebral pain on palpation together with muscle-tonic and neuro-reflex syndromes were recorded. Meningeal signs were absent.

The results of the neuropsychological and psychological tests are presented in Table 11.1. It is evident that the mental state of combatants was

Table 11.1 Neuropsychological and psycho/pathological examinations in ATO combatants (n = 54), control subjects, and comparison groups

Test	ATO combatants (n = 54) [M±SD]	Control group (n = 139) [M±SD]	Irradiated in utero and at age 0–1 years (n = 189) [M±SD]	Liquidators (n = 81) [M±SD]	Evacuees from Chernobyl exclusion zone (n = 76) [M±SD]	Afghan War veterans (n = 28) [M±SD]
MMSE	26.7±2.4	28.5±2.1*	27.8±2.8	25.6±2.9	26.1±2.4	25.7±2.6
GHQ–28	24.6±14.9	15.4±11.2*	20.4±11.2	41.4±12.4*	37.5±14.3*	29.7±13.3
SRDS	44.1±12.8	38.1±9.6	42.5±10.1	58.6±12.6*	56.9±11.7	47.8±12.6
IDA	3.7±3.4	1.9±1.9*	3.1±2.3	6.6±2.7*	5.4±2.4	4.8±2.5
IES	19.6±10.6	3.8±5.4*	4.4±5.4*	28.0±8.1*	25.6±5.5*	26.7±6.8*
M–PTSD	88.9±15.8	72.1±11.9*	86.4±16.5	99.9±17.4*	93.9±14.6	91.9±17.4

ATO = antiterrorism; GHQ–28 = General Health Questionnaire–28; IDA = Irritability, Depression, Anxiety Scale; IES = Impact of Events Scale; MMSE = Mini-Mental State Examination; M–PTSD = Mississippi Scale for Combat-Related PTSD; SD = standard deviation; SRDS = Self-Rating Depression Scale. According to the Bonferroni's correction, differences were considered to be significant at p <0.001. *Significantly different compared with the study group (ATO combatants), p <0.001.

significantly worse than that of control subjects, with more severe manifestations of PTSD, low health self-esteem, somatic concerns, anxiety, sleep–wake cycle disruptions, depression, social dysfunction, and mild cognitive impairment.

ATO combatants tended to have a better mental state than Afghan War veterans or the liquidators and evacuees from the Chernobyl exclusion zone. In particular, they showed a more appropriate emotional perception of the traumatic event. Their mental status was almost similar to that of the comparison group exposed to trauma during early development.

The personality profiles of the study group before ATO participation (assessed retrospectively) and at the time of examination showed marked personality deformations, revealing significantly ($p<0.001$) reduced extraversion, hyperthymia, increased neuroticism, jams, pedantry, excitability, dysthymia, and cyclothymia (see Figure 11.2).

Significant changes in cerebral brain activity, probably organic in nature, with bilateral paroxysmal activity, and increased spectral power in the beta range and decreased in the alpha range as revealed by qEEG, were detected only in ATO combatants.

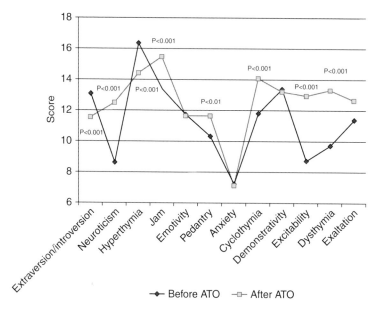

Figure 11.2. Profiles of personality before and after ATO participation.

Ultrasonic duplex scanning of the extracranial parts of the brachiocephalic vessels showed a thickening of the intima media in ATO combatants older than 50 years, while patients with commotio cerebri were characterized by venous dyshemia in the basal veins of Rosenthal.

The results of our clinical diagnoses of the study group are presented in Table 11.2. The main diagnoses were PTSD (91 per cent) and commotio cerebri (50 per cent). Also common were cervicalgia and lumbago, somatoform dysfunction of the autonomic nervous system, consequences of acoustic barotrauma, and conductive and sensorineural hearing loss. Several combatants suffered from comorbid somatic disorders. The syndrome of alcohol dependence was found in a small number of patients, mainly those from the armed forces (15 per cent).

Table 11.2 Clinical diagnoses according to the ICD–10 criteria in ATO combatants ($n = 54$)

Diagnosis	Absolute number	Relative-number
Neuropsychiatric symptoms/disorders	49	90.7
Posttraumatic stress disorder, F43.1	27	50.0
Commotio cerebri after ATO, S06.0	20	37.0
Cervicalgia, M54.2	16	29.6
Vegetative dystonia (somatoform dysfunction of autonomous nervous system), F45.3	13	24.1
Lumbago, M54.3; M54.4; M54.5	11	20.4
State after mine-blast acoustic barotrauma, T70.0	8	14.8
Chronic conductive and sensorineural hearing loss, H90.6	7	13.0
Acute conductive and sensorineural hearing loss, H90.6	6	11.1
Dyscirculatory encephalopathy (chronic ischemia of the brain, I67.8)	5	9.3
Alcohol dependence syndrome, F10.2	5	9.3
Adjustment disorder, F43.2	3	5.6
Stuttering (stammering), F98.5	1	2.0

Table 11.2 (cont.)

Diagnosis	Absolute number	Relative-number
Asthenic-vegetative syndrome (neurasthenia), (F48.0), accentuation of personality traits (Z73.1)	1	2.0
Cyst of transparent membrane of the brain, Q04.6	1	2.0
Arachnoidal cyst of the left temporal lobe, Q04.6	1	2.0
Retrocerebral arachnoidal cyst, Q04.6	1	2.0
Kimmerle anomaly, G99.2	1	2.0
Pineal gland cyst, D35.4	1	2.0
Condition after surgery (open head injury, S01)	1	2.0
Physical diseases		
Chronic ischemic heart disease, I25	12	22.2
Retinal vascular angiopathy, H31.8	11	20.4
Cholelithiasis, K80	8	14.8
Other nontoxic goiter, E04	6	11.1
Hypertensive heart disease, I11	4	7.4
Chronic gastritis and duodenitis, K29	4	7.4
Mitral (valve) prolapse, I34.1	2	3.7
Acute sinusitis, J01	2	3.7
Gastric, duodenal ulcer, K25, K26	2	3.7
Cardiomyopathy, I42	1	2.0
Other hypothyroidism, E03	1	2.0

Patients may show more than one diagnosis (all suffered from about four neuropsychiatric plus one physical diagnoses). ATO = antiterrorism; ICD–10 = International Statistical Classification of Diseases and Related Health Problems, 10th revision.

The empirical treatment of ATO combatants was based on pharmaco-therapy, including antidepressants (sertraline, escitalopram, amitriptyline, S-adenosyl-methionine); benzodiazepine (gidazepam) and non-benzodiazepine tranquilizers (hydroxyzine, aphobazolum, phenybutum); neuroprotective and vasoactive drugs (nicergoline, citicolinum, cortexin, cerebrolysin, actovegin, cavinton); and antiinflammatory and analgesic drugs (e.g., ibuprofen, diclophenac). Individual psychotherapy, eye move-ment desensitization and reprocessing, Erickson's therapy with hypnotic effect, neurolinguistic programming with training of control over one's emotional state, cognitive behavioral therapy, and/or positive psychother-apy were employed in combination with pharmacological treatments.

Discussion and Conclusions

The aim of our study was to assess the psychological and neuropsychiatric characteristics of 54 ATO combatants and to compare them with other subject groups: individuals exposed in utero at the time of the Chernobyl disaster; Chernobyl cleanup workers suffering from PTSD and comorbid chronic cerebrovascular pathology; subjects evacuated from the Chernobyl exclusion zone suffering from PTSD and comorbid chronic cerebrovascular pathology; and veterans of the Afghan War with PTSD following a closed head injury. Our results demonstrated that ATO combatants were characterized by low health self-estimation, somatic concerns, a high prevalence of PTSD, anxiety, insomnia, depression, social dysfunction, mild cognitive impairment, and neurological soft signs. In these respects, ATO combatants were quite similar to both the individuals involved in the Chernobyl disaster and the Afghan War veterans. Cervicalgia and lumbago, somatoform dysfunction of the autonomic nervous system, the consequences of acoustic barotrauma, and conductive and sensorineural hearing loss were also common.

Quantitative EEG showed abnormalities suggestive of irritation of the corticolimbic system and diencephalic structures. Ultrasonic duplex scanning of extracranial parts of the brachiocephalic vessels showed intima media thickening among ATO combatants older than 50 years of age and venous dyshemia in the basal veins of Rosenthal in patients with commotio cerebri.

Interestingly, personality changes were recorded retrospectively before as well as after armed conflict—in particular, while ATO combatants before the conflict showed extraversion and hyperthymia, upon returning home they demonstrated increased neuroticism, jams, pedantry, excitability, dysthymia, and cyclothymia.

The care of ATO combatants was based on a comprehensive approach including pharmacological/psychopharmacological drugs and different psychological techniques and psychotherapies. Although ours is an ongoing study, the preliminary data would suggest that this approach might be clini-cally very effective (data not shown).

The armed conflict in the Donbass is characterized by specific geopolitical and sociopsychological features. (1) It is a hybrid war within one nation state, Ukraine, which provokes the ethnocultural and sociopsychological characteristics of the "Donbass syndrome," with predominant severe social frustration and destruction of old relationships. (2) There are different kinds of populations involved in the conflict (ATO combatants, internal refugees and migrants, inhabitants of the occupied territories). (3) In the area where the antiterrorism campaign is being conducted (the temporarily occupied territories of the Donbass), there are many dangerous radioactive objects that could be used in terrorist attacks or, as a result of the fighting, present the danger of accidents caused by improper use and faulty maintenance. (4) There are many pregnant women and children who are among the groups of internally displaced persons and residents of the occupied territories. The armed conflict undoubtedly negatively affects the psychological and physical development of children.

The scope and affected populations of the armed conflict in the Donbass are more similar to those of the victims of the Chernobyl disaster and its aftermath than to other local military conflicts. It would certainly be worthwhile to try to overcome the medical and social consequences of the Donbass crisis based on our 30 years of experience with the consequences of the Chernobyl disaster and the related development by the NRCRM of systematic measures for mental healthcare following radiation accidents at nuclear reactors, terrorist attacks using a radiological dispersive device ("dirty bomb"), or the use of tactical nuclear weapons.[30–32]

As emphasized almost 25 years ago,[33] the key point in protecting the mental and physical health of those involved in traumatic emergencies is freedom of choice when it comes to risk. The results of our study confirm this opinion. The mental state of the surveyed ATO combatants is better than that of the liquidators and Afghan War veterans. Of course, much more time has passed since the Chernobyl disaster and the war in Afghanistan, compared to the trauma suffered by our ATO veterans. However, it should be underlined that most of the surveyed ATO participants were members of volunteer battalions. Therefore, the better mental state of the ATO combatants could be reasonably explained by their conscious and voluntary choice to accept the risks of war. In addition, volunteers from NGOs are likely to also play a significant role in supporting and maintaining the mental health of ATO combatants.

The present research is just a pilot study. However, combining the results of several decades of experience in facing and overcoming the health and social consequences of the Chernobyl disaster and our many years of neuropsychiatric research with war veterans, we feel confident in endorsing our scientific and organizational approaches to mental healthcare for ATO combatants, refugees, and migrants from the Donbass, which perhaps could be useful in other current conflicts.

The following guidelines are suggested

1. Voluntary participation and awareness of risk should be required for engagement in hostilities.

2. Accurate and stringent professional selection of special contingents (military and other security forces, rescue workers) based on stability of mental activity, a sthenic personality, and resistance to stress.

3. An adequate information policy: true, meaningful, and timely coverage of the current situation by the media (as well as online sources).

4. Panic prevention, detection, and isolation of elements that induce panic.

5. Formation of psychological and psychiatric teams with special skills. Crews are now working closely with ATO headquarters, local authorities, and health services (e.g., ambulance corps, specialized mental health facilities).

6. Preventive, sanitary, and educational work concerning risk management of mental disorders, especially regarding the harm of psychoactive substance use in emergencies.

7. Permanent active monitoring of the mental health of soldiers and settlers for early detection of mental and behavioral disorders and provision of evacuation.

8. Use of the maximal approach ("as close as possible") of psychological and psychiatric care in the theater of military operations and among immigrants.

9. An awareness that there is an increased risk of mental/behavioral disorders in those who need the most attention: the chronically mentally ill, the elderly and very elderly, children, and (especially pregnant) women.

10. Active engagement of religious and community organizations, volunteers, and local communities in providing psychological and psychiatric care.

11. Creation of a network of crisis and psychological rehabilitation centers and unification of the interdepartmental psychological/psychiatric areas.

12. Creation of special scientific and practical departments for emergency psychological and psychiatric care (emergency centers), as well as neuropsychiatric and mental rehabilitation centers within the structure of multidisciplinary hospitals/research centers and institutions.

13. Spa treatment and mental rehabilitation.

Implementation of the proposed approaches would constitute a significant and concrete step toward adequate mental healthcare for ATO combatants, refugees, and migrants from the Donbass, thus strengthening the capabilities and security of Ukraine, and perhaps those of other conflict areas.

Disclosures

Konstantin Loganovsky, Natalia Zdanevich, Marina Gresko, Donatella Marazziti, and Tatiana Loganovskaja hereby declare that they do not have anything to disclose.

References

1. Davidenkov, SN, ed. Neurological diseases (peculiarities of their origin, course, prevention and treatment during the war) [in Russian]. In: *The Experience of Soviet Medicine in the Great Patriotic War of 1941–1945, Part 2: Therapy*, **Vol. 26**, §10. Moscow: Medgiz; 1949: 55–91.

2. Kessler, RC, Üstün, TB, eds. The WHO World Mental Health Surveys: Global Perspectives on the Epidemiology of Mental Disorders. New York, NY: Cambridge University Press; 2008. Available at: assets.cambridge.org/97805218/84198/front matter/9780521884198_frontmatter.pdf.

3. World Health Organization. Guidelines for the Management of Conditions Specifically Related to Stress. Geneva: World Health Organization; 2013. Available at: http://apps.who.int/iris/bitstream/10665/85119/1/9789241505406_eng.pdf.

4. Steel, Z, Chey, T, Silove, D, Marnane, C, Bryant, RA, van Ommeren, M. Association of torture and other potentially traumatic events with mental health outcomes among populations exposed to mass conflict and displacement. *JAMA*. 2009; **302**(5): 537–549.

5. World Health Organization. World Health Report 2001. *Mental Health: New Understanding, New Hope*. Geneva: World Health Organization; 2001. Available at: www.who.int/whr/2001/en/whr01_en.pdf?ua=1.

6. Stratta, P, de Cataldo, S, Bonanni, R, Valenti, M, Masedu, F, Rossi, A. Mental health in L'Aquila after the earthquake. *Ann Ist Super Sanita*. 2012; **48**(2): 132–137. Available at: www.iss.it/publ/anna/2012/2/482132.pdf.

7. Bromet, EJ. Emotional consequences of nuclear power plant disasters. *Health Phys*. 2014; **106**(2): 206–210. Available at: www.ncbi.nlm.nih.gov/pmc/articles/PMC3898664/.

8. Legha, RK, Solages, M. Child and adolescent mental health in Haiti: developing long-term mental health services after the 2010 earthquake. *Child Adolesc Psychiatr Clin N Am*. 2015; **24**(4): 731–749. Epub ahead of print Jul 8.

9. Napryeyenko, OK, Syropyatov, OG, Druz, OV, et al. *Psychological and Psychiatric Assistance to Victims of Armed Conflicts (Guidelines)* [in Ukrainian]. Kyiv: Ministry of Public Health of Ukraine; 2014.

10. Napryeyenko, OK, Loganovsky, KM, Napryeyenko, NY, Loganovskaya, TK. Scientific support of non-governmental organizations of psychiatrists, narcologists and medical psychologists activities in Ukraine. *Clin Neuropsychiatry.* 2015; **12**(2): 23–26.

11. Bogomolets, OV, Pinchuk, IY, Druz, OV, et al. *Approaches of Optimization for Mental Health Care According to Current Needs of Participants of Military Actions (Guidelines)* [in Russian]. Kyiv: Ministry of Public Health of Ukraine, Ministry of Defence of Ukraine, Ukrainian Center of Scientific Medical Information and Patent License Activities; 2014.

12. Voloshin, PV, Maruta, NO, Shestopalova, LF, et al. *Diagnosis, Treatment and Prevention of Medical and Psychological Consequences of Combat Operations in Modern Conditions (Guidelines)* [in Ukrainian]. Kharkiv: Ministry of Public Health of Ukraine, National Academy of Medical Sciences of Ukraine, Ukrainian Center of Scientific Medical Information and Patent License Activities; 2014.

13. Kolesnik, M. Posttraumatic stress disorder: diagnostic, therapy, rehabilitation [in Ukrainian]. *Ukr Med J.* 2015; **4**(108): 8–10.

14. Moroz, SM, Makarova, II, Semenikhina, VE, et al. Phytoneuroregulation opportunity in patients with anxiety-depressive disorders as a result of military stress [in Russian]. *Ukr Med J.* 2015; **4**(108): 60–62.

15. Khaustova, OO, Kovalenko, NV. Current problems of life and mental health disorders in internally displaced persons [in Ukrainian]. *Arch Psychiatry.* 2015; **2** (81): 42–47.

16. Kochin, IV. Features of medical and sanitary losses and emergency medical care organization for population and military personnel in the area of anti-terrorist operations [in Ukrainian]. *News Med Pharm Ukr.* 2015; **14**(52): 16–18.

17. Tabachnikov, SI, Osukhovska, OS, Kharchenko, YM, et al. Sociodemographic and clinical psychopathological characteristics of psychoactive substance use, comorbid with PTSD, in the combatants of antiterrorist operation in Ukraine [in Ukrainian]. *Arch Psychiatry.* 2015; **21**(3–4): 82–83.

18. Kutko, II, Panchenko, OA, Linev, AN. Posttraumatic stress disorder in people suffering from armed conflict: clinical development, diagnostics, treatment and rehabilitation [in Russian]. *Ukr Med J.* 2016; **1**(111): 24–27.

19. World Health Organization. International Statistical Classification of Diseases and Related Health Problems, 10th rev. Vol. 2: Instruction Manual. Geneva: World Health Organization; 2010. Available at: www.who.int/classifications/icd/ICD10 Volume2_en_2010.pdf.

20. Folstein, MF, Folstein, SE, McHugh, PR. "Mini-Mental State": A practical method for grading the cognitive state of patients for the clinician. *J Psychiatr Res.* 1975; **12** (3): 189–198.

21. Goldberg, D. *The General Health Questionnaire: GHQ–28.* London: National Foundation for Educational Research–Nelson; 1981.

22. Goldberg, DP, Gater, R, Sartorius, N, et al. The validity of two versions of the GHQ in the WHO study of mental illness in general health care. *Psychol Med.* 1997; **27**(1): 191–197.

23. Shafer, AB. Meta-analysis of the factor structures of four depression questionnaires: Beck, CES–D, Hamilton, and Zung. *J Clin Psychol.* 2006; **62**(1): 123–146.

24. Horowitz, M, Wilner, N, Alvarez, W. Impact of the Event Scale: a measure of objective stress. *Psychosom Med.* 1979; **41**(3): 209–218.

25. Keane, TM, Caddell, JM, Taylor, KL. Mississippi Scale for Combat-Related Posttraumatic Stress Disorder: three studies in reliability and validity. *J Consult Clin Psychol.* 1988; **56**(1): 85–90.

26. Loganovsky, KN, Zdanevich, NA. Cerebral basis of post-traumatic stress disorder following the Chernobyl disaster. *CNS Spectr.* 2013; **18**(2): 95–110. Epub ahead of print Feb 27.

27. Schmieschek, H. Questionnaire for the Determination of Accentuated Personalities [in German]. *Psychiatr Neurol Med Psychol (Leipz).* 1970; **22**(10): 378–381.

28. Eysenck, HJ, Eysenck, SBG. *Manual of the Eysenck Personality Questionnaire.* London: Hodder and Stoughton; 1975.

29. Loganovsky, K, Gresko, M. *Personality Changes in Participants of Anti-Terrorist Operations in the Donbass and in Chernobyl Accident Survivors.* Paper presented at the International Conference on "Health Effects of the Chernobyl Accident—30-year Aftermath," April 18–19, 2016. Geneva: World Health Organization; Kyiv: National Academy of Medical Sciences of Ukraine and National Research Center for Radiation Medicine; 2016.

30. Loganovsky, KN, Bomko, MA, Chumak, SA. Scientific justification of the mental health system in radiation emergency situations (on the experience of the Chernobyl disaster) [in Russian]. *Psychiatry, Psychother Clin Psychol.* 2012; **2**(08): 20–36.

31. Loganovsky, KN, Chumak, SA, Bomko, MA. Mental health care and psycho-rehabilitation in radiation emergency situations (on the experience of the Chernobyl disaster) [in Russian]. *Emerg Med.* 2012; **2**(12): 75–106.

32. Loganovsky, KM, Petrychenko, OO, Morozov, OM, et al. *Mental Health Care in Radiation Accidents at Nuclear Reactors and the Using of "Dirty Bombs" and Tactical Nuclear Weapons (Guidelines)* [in Ukrainian]. Kyiv: Ministry of Public Health of Ukraine, Ministry of Defense of Ukraine, Ukrainian Center of Scientific Medical Information and Patent License Activities; 2014.

33. Niagu, AI, Noshchenko, AG, Loganovskii, KN. Late effects of psychogenic and radiation factors of the accident at the Chernobyl nuclear power plant on the functional state of the human brain [in Russian]. *Zh Nevropatol Psikhiatr Im S S Korsakova.* 1992; **92**(4): 72–77.

The International Scenario of Terrorism

Donato Marzano

12

The last century has been characterized by several events that have deeply influenced the geopolitical scenario and the evolution of modern society. Aside from natural events, the First and Second World Wars shaped international equilibrium. At the price of millions of deaths, Western societies, since the end of the 1940s, have begun a virtuous path to peace, paying attention to the industrial reconstruction, which in the postwar period represented exceptional support for the economies of the defeated nations. Despite all of this, the world soon became divided between two superpowers, the United States and the Union of Soviet Socialist Republics, and for this reason for four decades the global balance of power was unstable. The Cold War was a simmering conflict that created global suspense: a prolonged period that witnessed an indirect conflict between these two countries through distanced client wars, trying to affirm and promote opposite values and ideologies. This bipolar period was also characterized as the two sides "playing by the rules"— clear, precise, and binding, a dispute where the enemy was well-defined. The two superpowers established limits on the tensions born from other regional crises, considering themselves arbiters among opponents aligned with one group or another. As a consequence, the armed forces of both blocks developed different war doctrines, oriented by the historical moment and the perceived threat.[1]

The fall of the Berlin Wall in 1989 reshaped the interests of Europe, which were gradually emancipated from the fear of a Russian invasion. Thus, a redefinition of the military structure as a whole took place because the commanders in chief became aware of their inadequacy to face the new challenges. The failure of the communist ideology had two consequences: (1) remodulation of the role of the military, which in the past included surveillance and nuclear and conventional deterrence; and (2) a growing confusion, especially related to new and unpredictable scenarios.

Meanwhile, since the 1970s, terrorist groups well-rooted in different European nations progressively abandoned their endogenous characteristics and adopted a transnational approach based on common ideologies. The Brigate Rosse (BR) in Italy, the Rote Armee Fraktion (RAF) in Germany, the Irish Republican Army (IRA) in Ireland, and the Euskadi Ta

Askatasuna (ETA) in Spain, in their own ways, shook the civil consciousness by pursuing military agendas dictated by various ideologies. Their common element was the fight against the institutions of the state. However, the rise of these groups (just a few examples of the terrorist galaxy) represented the beginning of a long season of violence and blood, which were confronted with individual strategies (which yielded various results) by each state.

The first escalation in terms of the visibility and efficiency of terrorism was represented by the appearance on the international scene of the Islamist group in the powderkeg of the Middle East. The first attack carried out by terrorists was the massacre at the Munich Olympics in 1972, when Fedayyin commandos from the Black September terrorist organization broke into the athletes' housing and killed two Israelis, leading to a firefight with German police that brought on the death of all the Israeli hostages.

The media exposure and consequent social effect inspired the rise and proliferation of other groups throughout the world. With the ancient contraposition of Sunni and Shia believers, the Middle East became the terror laboratory, an authentic school. Moreover, the process of decolonization in several African countries represented a threat due to the increase in the number of new hostile forces. In that scenario, while the bipolar contraposition of the superpowers still exists, despite the beginning of a new season characterized by the dialogue between East and West, antiterrorist defence is called upon to answer the new threat. Endogenous terrorism is reinforced by similar organizations located in other nations, assuming wider regional connotations and rendering more difficult the preventive and repressive actions of investigative institutions.

Through the Camp David Accords of 1978, the process of building peace in the Middle East changed thanks to the end of the state of war between Israel and Egypt. Nevertheless, this historical agreement left several crisis situations unsolved, first and foremost the Lebanese and Palestinian situations, both tightly linked to the dynamic of the Syrian regime, a very discussed topic these days. However, the Camp David Accords embraced an innovative opportunity for a military instrument. The Multinational Force and Observers represent the first experiment of a "coalition of the willing." Italy discovered its vocation for foreign military missions, earning appreciation for their first military intervention in Lebanon led by General Angioni. It was a fundamental step in the acquisition of efficacy and experience useful for the consequent mission in the Persian Gulf.[2]

However, Western nations are not the only peacekeeping actors. In fact, the Soviet Union in 1979 tried a military experiment by invading Afghanistan to overthrow President Amin and impose a government led by Babrak Karmal. Moscow never thought that this would become the "Soviet Vietnam." Taking into account their military superiority, the Kremlin planned a sort of blitzkrieg, absolutely sure that they were able to defeat the Afghan fighters. Needless to say, it was not that simple, and that gave the chance for Russian leaders to change their initial intentions and abandon the mission. Nevertheless, the international community is still paying a great price for that war. The Afghan resistance was supported by nations that had the intention to weaken the Soviet Union by prolonging this proxy war. The mujahidin received unexpected support from different external actors who supplied arms, training, and equipment. Once the Afghan conflict came to its conclusion, it left in its wake some groups of resistance fighters influenced by radical Islamist ideology. These terrorist groups were trained through specific techniques that caused great difficulties for the better-equipped military forces, especially thanks to their better knowledge of the hostile territory. It was the fatherland of Al Qaeda, who represented a new phenomenon within the international panorama. It is a transregional organization that is constantly spreading and growing, thanks to the spontaneous affiliation of terrorist groups that share their ideology and goals. This new actor arose in a specific historical moment characterized by the disaggregation of the Soviet Union and the rise of new crisis sites and such failed states as Somalia. Today these organizations appear as secondary actors, because terrorism is now most dramatically linked with the Islamic State (or Daesh). The real power of this organization comes from its extraordinary media savvy, not its military capabilities. Techniques of attack, settled in the European capitals, belong to the tradition of Al Qaeda. Their tactics are organized in a simple fashion, and their efficacy derives from their willingness to sacrifice their lives, following religious rules erroneously derived from Islamic precepts. The simplicity of their attacks is supported by obsessive media exposure, which greatly magnifies their real achievements. Due to the fact that some young Muslims, often born in the West, do not feel integrated in their societies and seek to find a sense of belonging in their ancient origins, the terrorists have a vast supply of recruits from which to draw.

Prevention and repression of terrorism require capabilities that need to be trained within a short period of time. For this reason, it is fundamental to draw on the experience of military professionals who worked in the area where terrorism was born. The asymmetric techniques of terrorist attacks used by insurgents have caused such a huge number of victims, our military has allied itself with those of other countries (some strange bedfellows). The analysis of techniques and tactics led us to an awareness that the best training, as well as the best equipment, have next to no influence against enemies who see death as the supreme sacrifice that will connect them with their god and transport them to paradise.[3]

Those scenarios have radically changed all the long-consolidated doctrines employed during the Cold War. The enemy is no longer conventional, and neither are their armaments. Our doctrines should be adaptive and predictive. It is upon this framework that intelligence work has its floor. Constant activity in making relationships and building multicultural acceptance constitute the anthropological approach to the "operative theatre." The challenge is continuous and multipolar. Conflicts are fought on mountains, in deserts, in Western capitals, and in cyberspace, a limitless expanse where hunting requires creativity, human innovation, and technical tools.

Nowadays, the military arm of industrialized nations is moving toward this dimension, where one cannot smell the fear of the war but where a loss can cost thousands of lives. We now almost look back at the Cold War with a melancholic nostalgia. Four decades ago, soldiers wearing a uniform were easily identifiable as the enemy. The paradox is that the old enemy and we now face the same threat.

Disclosures

Admiral Marzano has nothing to disclose.

References

1. Judt, T. *Postwar: A History of Europe since 1945*. New York, NY: The Penguin Press; 2005.

2. Howard, Lise Morje. *UN Peacekeeping in Civil Wars*. Cambridge: Cambridge University Press; 2008.

3. Lutz, James M, Lutz, Brenda J. *Global Terrorism*. London, New York, NY: Routledge; 2004.

| Chapter | Identification and Prevention of |

13

Identification and Prevention of Radicalization. Practice and Experiences with a Multidisciplinary Working Model

Dorte Sestoft

Background

It is well known that psychiatric patients are exposed to an increased risk in many different areas. These areas include increased risk of social decline,[1-3] increased mortality from suicide as well as somatic illnesses,[4,5] increased risk for comorbidity in the form of substance abuse,[6] increased risk of criminal victimization,[7] and increased risk of committing violent crimes.[8] From the clinician's perspective, it is likely that the risk factors interact in a synergetic way and leave the psychiatric patient extremely vulnerable. To enhance supportive efforts in a more focused and coordinated direction, a new working model between public sectors was introduced in Denmark in 2004.

Cooperation between the police, social services, and psychiatry is an important part of the daily work for these professions in most countries. However, the cooperation generally involves only two sectors at a time. There was no formal cooperation between the three sectors in Denmark until the implementation of the PSP (police, social services, psychiatry) cooperation.

In 2004, the three sectors in the municipality of Frederiksberg (a municipality in the greater Copenhagen area with a total of 90,000 inhabitants) decided to intensify their cooperation to ensure that relevant information was shared and supportive measures enhanced concerning citizens at risk. The local police department, social services, and psychiatry/mental health services developed a new cooperation model: PSP cooperation.

On April 1, 2009, an act of Parliament scaled up the PSP cooperation to national coverage, and an evaluation of the cooperation was performed. The 2011 evaluation report stated that the PSP cooperation helped to highlight marginalized citizens at risk. It noted that, prior to PSP cooperation, authorities often lost focus on this population. The evaluation further reported, for example, that after the PSP implementation, there were fewer mentally ill people mentioned in police reports, fewer evictions, fewer domestic violence emergency calls, and generally improved cooperation between the sectors involved.[9] A detailed description of the PSP model and practice was published in 2014.[10]

Within the last few decades, radicalization and the threat of terrorism have become key issues in Denmark and many other societies. The Radicalization Awareness Network (RAN) was created by the European Commission in 2011 as a way of connecting first-line practitioners and local actors around Europe working with radicalization. Experiences from other European countries suggest that an interdisciplinary approach is central to the prevention of radicalization and the safeguarding of individuals at risk. Multi-agency co-operation seems necessary to provide a consistent and reliable network. Other EU countries have had promising experiences with multi-agency programs, including, for example, Community Policing and the Prevention of Radicalisation (CoPPRa) in Belgium, and Working with Potentially Violent Loners (PVL) in the Care Sector in the Netherlands.[11] RAN has, among many other initiatives, led to an increased focus on how employees in various governmental sectors react to concerns of possible radicalization among the citizens they meet or hear about through their work. From its beginnings in 2004, the three core sectors in the PSP cooperation have facilitated the identification of citizens at risk (e.g., of suicide, substance abuse, social decline, or mental illness) and coordinated the relevant intervention and treatment. Even though the literature does not link group-based terrorism to mental disorders, terrorists who act alone are more likely to have a background that includes mental illness.[12] The vulnerable psychiatric patient would be an easy target for radicalization, and hence, radicalization could be added to the long list of risk factors acquired with major mental illness. Therefore, the pre-existing PSP cooperation was an obvious forum for identifying and dealing with concerns about radicalization and extremism,[13] and the model is an example of an initiative that extends beyond criminal justice and includes public health policy and practice, which Weine et al.[14] describe as a capable approach.

Considerations about Why Radicalization becomes a Mental Health Issue

Based on clinical experience, different mechanisms can lead to radicalization among mentally ill patients. Radicalization can be a consequence of psychotic symptoms. Paranoid patients often use contemporary themes as a substrate for their delusions. Clinicians know that the number of Jesus Christs among psychotic patients increases significantly in the weeks before Christmas. It is, therefore, not surprising that exposure to extremism in the press and on the internet can result in delusions about being selected to a special mission or paranoid delusions about surveillance.

Moreover, being a psychiatric patient is often associated with loss of social and daily life skills as well as cognitive difficulties leading to a decline of expectation of life possibilities. This could leave the patient in a lonely, marginalized, or even excluded position, the same position many young people from ethnic minorities feel that they are in—even though their paths are quite different.

Vignette 1: J was an elderly woman suffering from schizophrenia. She was very ambivalent about her illness and treatment, and she isolated herself from family and friends. She contacted a totally unknown imprisoned man sentenced for Islamist terrorism and started visiting him. Shortly later, she converted to Islam and changed her name, habits, and dress code. She now felt that she had a new belonging. After a few months, she contacted a staff member because she had concerns about things she was asked to do, and she wanted help and protection to step back from the relationship.

PSP and the Danish Prevention Approach, the Role of the Danish Security and Intelligence Service (PET) and the "Info-house Concept"

Since the middle of this century's first decade, there has been an increasing focus on countering violent extremism (CVE) as a supplement to the more traditional counterterrorism measures. The so-called "home-grown terrorists" posed a new threat to society. Therefore, the Danish Security and Intelligence Service (PET) changed its focus from a political security agenda to include a national social focus and, thereby, cooperate with local crime-prevention collaboration networks.

The Danish prevention approach is rooted in two areas of concern: the protection of the state and society against terrorist attacks, and the welfare state's responsibility for the individual's well-being. This protects the individual against self-harming behavior and engaging in crime, including terrorist-related offences—the so-called "Danish model."[15,16]

Thus, the prevention of radicalization and violent extremism has been incorporated into the existing prevention methods and structures, now also including the PSP model, with radicalization becoming another parameter of concern for the ordinary prevention system. The PSP cooperation facilitates cooperation and information-sharing between the different authorities with the aims of protecting society from crime and preventing individuals from engaging in crime, including violent extremism. This means that the PSP is aware of an individual's risk of radicalization on the same level as other types of risk behavior.

Since 2009, so-called Info-houses have been established in all 12 Danish police districts. They encompass a formal structure or network of local professionals from different sectors working in the field of CVE. It is expedient for all stakeholders to have a formal forum where local challenges and concrete concerns related to radicalization can be discussed. It also enables a clear distribution of duties and responsibilities that can be initiated from the outset, avoiding cases being lost or neglected in referrals from one authority to another.

When considered relevant, the Info-house can refer cases to the existing local prevention collaboration networks in which the police and the municipality also participate, that is, the PSP cooperation. Thus, appropriate actions can be taken in a rapid, effective, and coordinated manner. Because challenges with crime, including radicalization and violent extremism, frequently cut across municipal boundaries, a strength of the Info-house is the horizontal connection whereby different municipalities in the police district can solve challenges together. Finally, it is possible for the PET to pass on cases to the Info-house for rehabilitative measures which local authorities should administer.

Structured Cooperation as a Platform for Dealing with Concerns of Radicalization

Incorporating radicalization awareness into the PSP model renders it possible for the psychiatric system to bring a concern to the formal forum where local challenges and concrete concerns related to radicalization can be discussed. In the PSP forum, a concrete concern coming from, for instance, the psychiatric sector can be brought up and discussed, and if the police officers who are specially trained to recognize and deal with concerns of radicalization agree that there is an actual concern based on their knowledge of the individual, they can refer the case to the Info-house. When the Info-houses receive a report of possible radicalization, they conduct a more thorough assessment of whether these concerns are warranted. If they find that there are grounds for concern, they assess whether this is primarily related to and best dealt with as a social challenge, or whether there are security aspects.

When PET's Prevention Center receives a report of possible radicalization, they conduct an intelligence-led assessment. If this assessment evidences that there is no threat to national security, but there is still a case of radicalization risk, the case is referred back to the Info-house for rehabilitation measures. PET offers advice on which rehabilitation measures should be used by the local authorities through the Info-house. Moreover, this model also renders it possible for the police and/or PET to refer cases from the police system into a treatment system (Figure 13.1).

Training Courses Aimed at PSP Cooperation Professionals

To upgrade the skills of the PSP cooperation employees regarding how to handle concerns about radicalization in their daily work, the Danish Agency for International Recruitment and Integration (SIRI) and PET organized a two-day course beginning in 2013 for all PSP groups on a national level.

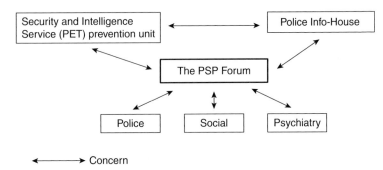

Concern

Figure 13.1. PSP and radicalization awareness. The figure illustrates how concerns can be shared and discussed within the different sectors. The PSP forum is the central platform. PSP can receive concerns about radicalization from front-line workers in all three sectors. It can also receive concerns from above, for example, the Security and Intelligence Service (PET). PSP can also share concerns with the relevant counterpart.[13]

These courses aimed to raise the awareness of radicalization among the PSP network and provide the attendees with knowledge of radicalization as a social, psychological, and political phenomenon. The courses aimed to give the participants knowledge of the Danish model, strategy, and methods for preventing radicalization in general and among mentally vulnerable people. Moreover, the courses also aimed to inform participants about the "standard operating procedure" within the organization and communication tools when dealing with concerns over possible radicalization.

The focus of the training was to ensure proportionality in the handling of cases, emphasizing that the measures taken must match the risk. Furthermore, the courses addressed the risk of stigmatization, focusing on the importance of cases being handled by the PSP collaboration rather than PET to avoid this concern. It is important to stress that the cooperation between PET and the PSP system goes both ways; the primary aim being to help individuals at risk.

Following the training session, SIRI was responsible for evaluating the outcome in close cooperation with PET and the Ministry of Health. An external consulting agency, EPINION, carried out the evaluation.[17] The assessment ran from October 2014 through December 2016 and covered the degree of benefit and the usefulness of the radicalization prevention course aimed at professionals from the three PSP sectors.

The evaluation took place in two parts. First was a quantitative study based on a survey including all participants, who completed a questionnaire immediately after the course and a follow-up after six months. Second was a qualitative interview study based on interviews with 20 relevant professionals in the PSP organization regarding both the steering and operational levels.

Staff Evaluation of the Initiative

The evaluation of the upgrading of the employees in the PSP cooperation was published in 2017. It was based on a survey eliciting 249 responses done shortly after the course and a follow-up survey done after six months and eliciting 181 responses. Overall, the course was assessed positively. The course contributes to important knowledge in relation to radicalization and extremism. Before the course, 35 per cent of the participants assessed that they had a good or extensive knowledge of radicalization and extremism. After the course, 95 per cent of the participants assessed this to be the case. The evaluation shows that the course contributes to an increased focus on radicalization and extremism in the participants' daily work. About nine of 10 participants report that this is the case. Regarding practical utility, more than half of the participants assess that they have been able to apply knowledge and new tools in their work. One-third of the participants have dealt with at least one case of concerns about extremism or radicalization six months after the course and 13 per cent more than one case.[17]

Does PSP Cooperation Prevent Radicalization on the Case Level?

There has not yet been a formal evaluation of the referred cases. However, seen from a national-security perspective, there is every indication that the use of the PSP cooperation as a platform for handling concerns about radicalization and violent extremism is effective.

The PET has addressed cases in which mental illness was considered a major contributing cause of the threats that fall under PET's field of operation, including, for example, radicalization or threats to public individuals.

With the PSP collaboration, it is possible to refer suitable cases of this type to the mental health services. Here, the local PSP network can reduce the potential threat that the individual poses by focusing on the well-being of the individual through mental health treatment and support in their everyday life. Because a potential threat can be reduced by focusing on the person's well-being at the community level where preventive measures can be initiated, one of the results of using the PSP is that PET can potentially avoid implementing costly and more invasive traditional security and intelligence measures. Moreover, as illustrated in vignettes 2 and 3, the cooperation model also facilitates protection of vulnerable citizens from being pushed into radicalization by people close to them, for example, in their family or neighborhood.

The PSP cooperation can also be useful in relation to aftercare for returning foreign fighters. In some cases, returnees may have symptoms of, for example, post-traumatic stress disorder (PTSD), which can potentially increase the threat they pose to national security. If the treatment system deals with these symptoms, the level of the threat will potentially decrease. Thus, if there is a suspicion of psychiatric and/or psychological problems, the PSP collaboration can support rehabilitation measures in the disengagement process.

Finally, it is important to stress that cooperation between the different sectors and the PSP system goes both ways, with the primary aim of helping those who are at risk. Mentally ill people are particularly vulnerable in terms of being a danger to themselves and others; therefore, they are also particularly vulnerable to radicalization and, thus, at particular risk of being caught by extremism.

The following cases took place around the same time in a neighborhood visited by an assertive interdisciplinary psychiatric team in Denmark. The team provided intensive outpatient care to patients suffering mainly from schizophrenia. Being involved in the PSP network as a part of the inter-sectorial approach in Danish psychiatry, the police provided the team with knowledge of relevant criminal movement in the area and the PSP network was, among other things, used to qualify the patients' experiences. Assessments in the following cases were made based on close knowledge of the patients and qualified by the knowledge and tools provided through close cooperation with the police and social services.

Vignette 2: A man of Middle Eastern origin known by the team for years was often sitting in public talking and shouting while laughing out loud. Because of his odd behavior, he had had complaints from neighbors, and social services were working to provide supported housing for him. He began complaining about being sought out by what he described as extremist Muslim groups encouraging him to join them. He found it frustrating and worrisome, mostly because he was a liberal Muslim and found it difficult to reject them. This behavior was unusual for this particular patient, and thus, the team decided to take his complaints seriously and not write them off as delusional. Knowing him, he was closely monitored while working intensively on motivating him for admission to a psychiatric ward. The team supported him when he wanted to terminate his lease and worked closely with social services, and thus, he was provided supported housing in another part of town.

Vignette 3: A man of African descent suffering from schizophrenia was referred to the team. There was already a dialogue with social services about supported housing. The patient was complaining about being sought out by Muslim groups at home. He was very scared and suddenly decided to terminate his lease and became homeless. Thus, he went in and out of the psychiatric ward. He began making threats about getting a gun and shooting people. He was motivated for admission and the psychiatrist who admitted him contacted the local PSP cooperation for advice. The patient was not discharged until he could be placed in supported housing.

Conclusion

The formalized PSP cooperation is a promising platform for handling concerns about radicalization in order to facilitate prevention and intervention.

Acknowledgments

This chapter draws heavily on the co-authored paper "The police, social services, and psychiatry (PSP) cooperation as a platform for dealing with concerns of radicalization".[13] I thank my co-authors for allowing this.

I also thank social worker Laura Arendt for contributing with two of the vignettes presented here and Anne Groule, academic secretary, Ministry of Justice, Clinic of Forensic Psychiatry, Denmark, for her help in the process of preparing this chapter.

References

1. Nordt, C, Müller, B, Rössler, W, Lauber, C. Predictors and course of vocational status, income, and quality of life in people with severe mental illness: a naturalistic study. *Soc Sci Med.* 2007; **65**(7): 1420–1429. doi: 10.1016/j.socscimed.2007.05.024.

2. Miech, R, Caspi, A, Moffitt, TE, Wright, BRE, Silva, P. Low socioeconomic status and mental disorders: a longitudinal study of selection and causation during young adulthood. *Am J Sociol.* 1999; **104**(4): 1096–1131. doi: 10.1086/210137.

3. Dohrenwend, BP. Sociocultural and socio-psychological factors in the genesis of mental disorders. *J Health Soc Behav.* 1975; **16**: 365–392.

4. Nordentoft, M, Wahlbeck, K, Hällgren, J, et al. Excess mortality, causes of death and life expectancy in 270,770 patients with recent onset of mental disorders in Denmark, Finland and Sweden. *PLOS ONE.* 2013; **8**(1). doi: 10.1371/journal.pone.0055176.

5. Laursen, TM, Munk-Olsen, T, Gasse, C. Chronic somatic comorbidity and excess mortality due to natural causes in persons with schizophrenia or bipolar affective disorder. *PLOS ONE.* 2011; **6**(9). doi: 10.1371/journal.pone.0024597.

6. Toftdahl, NG, Nordentoft, M, Hjorthøj, C. Prevalence of substance use disorders in psychiatric patients: a nationwide Danish population-based study. *Soc Psychiatry Psychiatr Epidemiol.* 2016; **51**(1): 129–140. doi: 10.1007/s00127-015-1104-4.

7. Maniglio, R. Severe mental illness and criminal victimization: a systematic review. *Acta Psychiatr Scand.* 2009; **119**(3): 180–191. doi: 10.1111/j.1600-0447.2008.01300.x.

8. Honings, S, Drukker, M, ten Have, M, De Graaf, R, Van Dorsselaer, S, Van Os, J. Psychotic experiences and risk of violence perpetration and arrest in the general population: a prospective study. *PLOS ONE.* 2016; **11**(7): 1–17. doi: 10.1371/journal.pone.0159023.

9. Vitus, K, Kjær, AA. PSP-Samarbejdet – En kortlægning af PSP-Frederiksberg, Odense, Amager og Esbjerg; Report. 2011; ISBN: 9788771190090.

10. Sestoft, D, Rasmussen, MF, Vitus, K, Kongsrud, L. The police, social services and psychiatry cooperation in Denmark – a new model of working practice between governmental sectors. A description of the concept, process, practice and experience. *Int J Law Psychiatry.* 2014; 37(4): 370–375. doi: 10.1016/j.ijlp.2014.02.007.

11. RAN. RAN collection preventing radicalisation to terrorism and violent extremism; Report. 2017. https://ec.europa.eu/home-affairs/sites/homeaffairs/files/what-we-do/networks/radicalisation_awareness_network/ran-best-practices/docs/ran_collection-approaches_and_practices_en.pdf.

12. Royal College of Psychiatrists. Counter-Terrorism and Psychiatry. Position Statement; 2016; www.rcpsych.ac.uk/pdf/PS04_16.pdf.

13. Sestoft, D, Hansen, SM, Christensen, AB. The police, social services, and psychiatry (PSP) cooperation as a platform for dealing with concerns of radicalization. *Int Rev Psychiatry.* 2017; 29(4): 350–354. doi: 10.1080/09540261.2017.1343526.

14. Weine, S, Eisenman, DP, Kinsler, J, Glik, DC, Polutnik, C. Addressing violent extremism as public health policy and practice. *Behav Sci Terror Polit Aggress.* 2017; 9(3): 208–221. doi: 10.1080/19434472.2016.1198413.

15. Hemmingsen, AS. An introduction to the Danish approach to countering and preventing extremism and radicalization; 2015. www.ft.dk/samling/20151/almdel/reu/bilag/248/1617692.pdf.

16. The Danish Government. Preventing extremism and radicalisation policy; 2016; http://uim.dk/publikationer/preventing-and-countering-extremism-and-radicalisation/.

17. EPINION. Evaluering af kursusrække om radikalisering og ekstremisme; 2017. https://stopekstremisme.dk/filer/rapport-evaluering-af-kursusraekke-om-forebyggende-indsats-mod-radikalise.pdf.

How to Fight Terrorism? Political and Strategic Aspects

Erich Vad

Ideational Framework

Western societies have become accustomed to terrorism over the past 15 years. 9/11 opened a kind of "gate" for this phenomenon. Recent terrorist attacks have demonstrated the ever-growing and comprehensive vulnerability of Western societies, although terrorists have changed their structural and ideological faces since 9/11.

Terrorism sponsored by Al Qaeda and, gaining prominence in the past 4 to 5 years, Daesh, has become a global, border-transcending phenomenon. Salafists, another group of current relevance, includes some 10,000 followers, thousands of whom are prone to violence, as well as being ready and willing to act as terrorists. Taking our own interest into account, we must not put all Salafists under general suspicion. Certainly, it is not true that all European Salafists are sympathizing with terrorism. One thing we do know about is the phenomenon of returnees—persons who were involved in operations in the Middle East but, instead of remaining, returned to Europe. Many of them are deeply radicalized and show a high potential to engage in terrorist activities. I would like to stress the notion of "potential" as a caveat. Nevertheless, secret service findings and studies indicate that many of the recent assassins had a history of being fighters in Syria, Iraq, and Afghanistan. Others were radicalized by the intractable conflicts in these countries or inspired by the role model of radical fighters in these conflicts.

Terrorists who are inspired or even sponsored by Daesh or other radical organizations view Western states (with their open and democratic societies and their liberal way of life) as their key enemies. These terrorist groups are clearly aware of their military inferiority vis-à-vis Western military capabilities. For this reason, they are engaged in a long-term battle of attrition seeking the largest possible number of victims. It is not the quick fix, the short-term victory, which is their aim. Numerous smaller attacks on different targets is their approach to demoralizing Western societies. Those attacks have been organized in a decentralized manner, always more or less out of the blue, mostly unforeseeable, since decentralization provides terrorists with huge leverage over Western security forces. Terrorist groups are acting like the heads of a hydra. For this reason, eliminating a single element or even wiping out leading figures does not lead to a collapse of the overall organization. Decentralization works like protective gear and keeps up groups' striking capability.

Although not immediately apparent, terrorism forces us to take a stand and fight for our values. If we are not ready to do this, terrorism will be the trigger for the dissolution of our world and our way of life. Fighting terrorism is an existential matter for us. And it is *long past time* that we recognized this fact.

Fighting Root Causes and Prevention

Fighting terrorism requires a thorough and permanent analysis of the root and underlying causes. The results of those analyses form the basis for preventive measures. Various literature provides ample analysis on the root causes and underlying issues. For this reason, I will delve immediately into prevention.

Acting against Daesh in Iraq and Syria is directly related to domestic security and stability in our Western societies. Terrorist groups can follow migration routes or make use of them to distribute their ideology in recipient countries. This spreading of ideology is directly impacted by terrorist activities in conflict regions, which help to worsen tensions between ethnic and religious groups in Western countries.

Terrorism may contribute to radicalization in open, free, liberal, and democratic societies. Additionally, it may lead to social destabilization. On the domestic level, counterterrorism aims to minimize parallel societies, ghettos, no-go-areas, or problematic suburbs in major cities. Zero-tolerance programs and police forces who are adequately equipped and specialized seem a proper way to prevent home-grown terror cells. Additionally, people who live in those areas need alternative paths and perspectives to develop their lives. It is about solving the problem where it is rooted. In its essence, it is not about solving the problem in the country of import.

Social support needs to be done mainly within the framework of the Islamic community. They should be encouraged to assist in preventing radicalization. On the other hand, if those organizations become safe havens for terrorists, they have to be forbidden. For this reason, their logistic and financial flows from abroad have to be monitored. It is important to initiate public points of contact that are embedded. They serve as a link among governmental, federal, and communal authorities.

The key focus must be to socially ostracize terrorism and delegitimize it. We must try to separate terrorists from their safe havens and their supportive environment. They must not have any further safe havens for regeneration within our societies. There must not be intact options for recruitment via the internet. It is of essential importance to make the scope and brute force of terrorist attacks public, particularly via pictures. This is another way to delegitimize terrorism.

Parents, teachers, imams, street workers, and psychologists can be most valuable preventative assets. However, they must not be seen as agents of the state. This can lead to their delegitimation and can be counterproductive for counterterrorist efforts. Nevertheless, these community leaders and professional, who work at the microlevel, should also coordinate their efforts with security institutions in order to provide a more effective approach. It would be best to keep the relationship informal or discreet to avoid potential counterproductive effects.

Media and Social Networks

Social media such as Twitter and Facebook have been frequently used by terrorist organizations to spread their messages and ideas. Live streams of attacks are meant to gain additional attention in the broad public. There have even been virtual marketing campaigns launched by terrorist organizations. Particularly Daesh has become a perfect emulator. It produces and presents its footage as if it was a high-end Hollywood trailer. Terrorist organizations have found that a punchy picture is worth more than a thousand words.

It is a weird situation: both need each other, the media and terrorist organizations. This might be a provocative thesis, yet it is worth considering. The World Wide Web is open to everyone. It is open to all kinds of ideas, no matter whether they are supportive for the general public or destructive. Of course, it is always a matter of perspective and position when judging about supportive or not supportive. Yet, our preventive countermeasures must begin within social networks. This is crucial for influencing target groups about our agenda.

Current terrorism's target is to kill in the most brutal way to raise the threat and shock level among the general population to its maximum. Injured and bleeding victims on the road are not their target, but their means. The center of attention is the broader public—its insecurity and panic. For this reason, it takes pictures—from the sea front, from shopping centers, from Christmas markets, dead bodies lying around as a symbol of destruction, juxtaposing the summer atmosphere, shopping on a lazy Friday afternoon during the holiday season and, finally, just as a showcase, countering the pre-Christmas mood in one of Europe's largest cities.

What happened in the days after? Commentators and experts presented themselves on camera and talked about giving up some fundamental rights for the sake of security. For sure, nothing will change in the case of the next attack. Experts are amply available. Journalists and photographers are dependent on sensational news. The general public has to be fed, and it has the right to information. The system is bluntly beating itself with its own means.

Everybody plays their assigned part, often without being conscious of doing so. Of course, some know pretty well how to drive the public and how to make use of the mainstream and social media. No one is innocent. Recently a whole "industry of widespread concern" has appeared. And it is continuing to grow. It has become fashionable to "show social media concern." It is easy to express concern via Facebook, Twitter, and Instagram, etc. It is easy to quickly type some words or lines. It is easy to copy and paste a picture of concern. A new community of mourning and weeping has been emerging right after attacks. Compassion has become shallow. "Je suis" storms have become a new, short-lived phenomenon. What I am trying to express is a self-repeating situation with a kind of escalatory pattern.

Terrorism has become an extreme manner of communication and provocation. The media and means of communications are employed as weapons, airplanes in the case of 9/11, mostly in a self-repeating way.

I would go a step further. I claim that, without modern media, international terrorism in its current shape would not exist. Social media and media as such are key drivers in creating our political and societal reality. They offer pictures and narratives of terrorism, thereby spreading anxiety, shock, and awe. We participate in real time in the ongoing events as news agencies put terrorist attacks in the spotlight. This is exactly what terrorists want. The media plays an enhancing role. Indirectly or directly, they motivate broad spectrums of the public to mentally and psychologically take on the next chapter of the story. We are not only the audience and potential victims but also the culprits and actors. Modern terrorism is perfectly tailor-made for our media landscape. During the counterterrorist operations in France and Belgium in Brussels, the police had to ask the news agencies not to show pictures of ongoing operations. During the operation in January 2015 in Paris, the police could not storm the hostage-takers' hideaway since everything was on live TV. Terrorists often observe preparations by the police on TV or on the internet, which makes it easier for them to adapt their plans.

One could even say that terrorism and media are two sides of the same coin.[1] Journalists and the growing number of self-acclaimed "terror experts" are highly paid profiteers of terrorism. It is worthless and useless for terrorists if an attack is not broadly and extensively laid out and discussed in the media. Journalists and media cannot act differently. In fact, their hands are tied. They carry the message of terrorism on because they feel forced to tell what is going on. This is their job. And they thereby become the unwitting accomplices of terrorists.

Daesh produces highly professional texts, pictures, and videos each day.[2] Every terrorist organization has a team of media specialists. Success is measured by how long and how often the attack is reported in the news. The size of a headline in the print media is a measure of success. Success is judged by the importance attached to an attack.

At first glance, keeping an attack secret might seem to be the best solution to contain terrorism. Maybe it would be a means to push terrorism from our screens. Yet, we are living in the time of the internet, social media, and smartphones. They are the burgeoning realms of publication. Silencing an attack would open up space for conspiracy theories. Nevertheless, the media must not support the spread of fear and awe during and after terrorist attacks by promoting them and offering them broad coverage.

Some years ago, for instance, CNN showed videos of decapitations. Fox News broadcast a film of the burning of a Jordanian pilot on its website. None could explain the reasoning for doing so, apart from the sheer lust for sensation and, of course, expressing indignation afterwards.

What about the following: what if professional journalists would hesitate automatically for a moment before they spread news?

Speed has become a weak point in the media. One could even say that "speed kills." Professional journalists ask, "Cui bono if I spread the news? Do I contribute to the solution? Or do I become, even subconsciously, an accomplice of terrorism?" This might be the first step, a kind of positive self-restriction.

However, the media is driven by the principles of the free market, and the chances are that competing agencies would not act cooperatively to suppress sensationalism. It seems to be a solvable problem. For this reason, terrorism and media have a strong connection. Saying it even more bluntly: they are mutually complicit.

It is of utmost importance that our media develop an internationally accepted code of conduct. It has to include ways and means for how to deal with terrorism and what must not be done. Additionally, one could use social media consciously to prosecute terrorists.

Smartphone users may be asked to take part in the hunt for terrorists on the run. If a terrorist can meet everybody, at any time and at any place, why not turn the tables? Why not ask the public to support the police by providing informal information? It would provide the public with a feeling of at least doing something against terrorism and not being only a powerless victim. One could also search by means of digital profiling. We simply have to turn the tables and make use of the modern means of communication as an instrument of counterterrorism. Some ideas may involve a delicate balancing act between personal freedom and public safety, while others will be easy and even simple to implement. We must be proactive.

Who prevents us from digitalizing people by DNA profiling to simplify the fight against criminals and terrorists? Our freedom is much more challenged and endangered by international terror networks. Terrorists started to use the internet as a recruitment platform and to plan terrorist attacks a long time ago. Increasing security is not free of charge. If we want to fight terrorism successfully, we must take a huge and courageous "digital step."

Much will be new, simply because the existing frameworks and models do not work anymore.

Defeats as a New Training Ground

Defeats are not necessarily negative. To the contrary, a defeat in fighting terrorism can offer a series of alternatives on to-does, on not-to-does, and on alternative courses of action. Simply speaking, defeats, seen properly, could offer new training grounds as lessons identified and lessons learned.

When Palestinian terrorists took hostages during the Munich Olympic Games in 1972, none of the local authorities were prepared to react appropriately. German security forces were empty-handed. One of a number of consequences was the establishment of the GSG-9 counterterrorist unit. Some years later, this very unit was successfully and spectacularly freeing hostages in the wake of a plane hijacking in Mogadishu.

Numerous experiences such as the years-long fight against the Red Army Faction (RAF) or the rightwing group "NSU" have made the weak points in counterterrorism rather obvious.

In the meantime, a merciless competition between security authorities and terrorists is under way. The 9/11 attacks cost some hundreds of thousands of USD to carry out.[3] Renting or stealing a truck and using it as a lethal weapon is comparatively inexpensive—as witnessed in Nice, Berlin, and Stockholm.

It is obvious that terrorists inspire others to become terrorists and that their attacks show a certain pattern and share a number of commonalities. It seems to be a chain of unrelated and at the same time related attacks created by inspiration.

How do we deal with this phenomenon? Currently, there are no quick fixes close at hand. This is most likely the key issue related to the overall situation, providing a huge opportunity for those who are radically prone to exploit. It is virtually impossible to trace them in a reliable manner. For this reason, containment is wishful thinking, but there is no real option at the moment.

Terrorist groups have changed their face over the past 15 years. Al Qaeda-style attacks have morphed into homegrown terrorists and inspired groups without a direct link to Al Qaeda as such. The same may be said of Daesh. Recently, lone-wolf attackers have come to the public's attention. Yet, even if we follow the lone-wolf hypothesis, there is certainly a network of supporters and accomplices. Probably not in the classical sense, but there is certainly a strong ideational background. Lone-wolf attacks of larger scope are rarely spontaneous. They need thorough planning, organization, and logistics—even if it is a rather simple-appearing attack with trucks and handmade explosives. There is still a logistical chain, be it in a material way or in terms of being an inspiration.

At the same time, the internet provides many options to take action without causing a big stir. It is a rather complex and sometimes contradictory situation that we are confronted with. Of course, there are similarities between the terrorist attacks. Yet, they do not take the same patterns. That makes it more difficult to get hold of terrorists, since much develops and transpires beneath the surface.

One of the key challenges is fast radicalization via the internet and the unrestricted migration to Europe. The Wurzburg terrorist lived in Germany for months, without documents and without being checked by German authorities. His German host family did not think for a moment that they were giving room and board to a terrorist. External European borders are still open for everybody, and the fight against terrorism begins at the borders.

The 2011 Norwegian lone-wolf attacker misled security authorities for a long time before he did his murderous work. Security authorities stood on the sidelines, because action forces did not have the logistics for a quick and efficient counterattack.

Mumbai-style attacks (in 2008, 10 terrorists killed 170 and wounded hundreds in a hotel using automatic rifles) vividly demonstrated the police force's limitations. For this reason, it is of utmost importance to have a considerable number of high-quality and centrally located special forces. Centralization enables deployment via helicopter to hotspots.

Basically, each location must be reachable by reaction forces in a quick manner and at any point in time. Yet, this will not prevent terrorist attacks. Nevertheless, the secret services form the core for prevention of terrorist attacks.

Resilience Instead of Pacifism

Pacifism has a long tradition in the Western world.[4] Two world wars in the twentieth century and a population that has been deeply shaped by war form the background for pacifism in Europe. At the same time, a peaceful period of more the 70 years has created a number of generations that have never experienced the horrors of war. There is a mood of preserving the peace and at the same time being afraid of war that is shaping the attitude of many Europeans. Our social model, which offers considerable and comprehensive freedom, has created a mass of people who appreciate convenience, hedonism, liberalism, and all kinds of freedom (e.g., as laid down in the four freedoms by the European Union).

Now the liberal social model is at risk due to a number of issues, including terrorism, demographic change, economic issues, the re-emergence of nationalism, and a huge wave of refugees. Europe is no longer innocent.

So what to do? We do need resilience in our liberal, open, and democratic societies to counterbalance the new waves of terrorist violence. Resilience is a matter of changing the mindset of the population. There is definitely room for improvement and development.

Terrorism challenges us in an existential way, whether we want it to or not. Contrary to us, the terrorist loves to fight for life and death. He/she does not view us as a partner in dialogue and conflict. The only idea is to destroy our way of life. He/she is not afraid of death, but awaits it coolly. He/she is deploying life to destroy life. He/she seems to toss life away for a seemingly higher cause. He/she lives as a freedom fighter, bound by his/her worldview, and his/her religiosity, which makes her/him apparently unique.

This way of living stands in stark contrast to the primarily hedonist Western worldview. His/her approach provides him/her with a robust narrative. He/she has a distinctive personality. He/she exercises power over us by terror. He/she never learned to trust in borders so as to be able to live an acceptable life. He/she wants to be free in an archaic manner, by taking life and by putting his/her life at the disposal of a grand cause.

Friedrich Nietzsche may have offered an explanatory background to better understand what is going on. We, the Western world, was viewed by Nietzsche as the "last man." We live in societies that are shaped by materialism and self-interest. Our main focus is this world and the accumulation of material wealth. We may talk together and seem struck by terrorist events, but we lack deep social cohesion. If the fight against terrorism becomes too expensive, we are ready to give up. This attitude is well-known among terrorists, and this is one of the reasons why they scorn us so deeply. Moreover, terrorists force us to spend huge amounts of money on protection and countermeasures. This means that we do not have those resources available for other important issues and social concerns. Forced budgetary and resource redistributions change our societies. We are wealthy, rich, old, and weak.[5] We manage crises only within a framework of peaceful discourse and harmony that is free of domination. Supremacy leads us into internal and external capitulation and submission. We prefer to surrender instead of undertaking courageous steps. If we are confronted with brute force, we are concerned or even enraged—at worst.

The more an attack rocks the lives of people, the more our will is lessened to fight these opponents. Our religion is at its core hedonism, borderless personal self-fulfillment, and pure consumption. We cover our cowardice by calling it pacifism. We forget to fight for life and death. We cling to material goods much more than to our freedom. In actual fact, the Western mass democracies have basically lost their freedom. Everything has become like a supermarket, stuffed with worldviews and different narratives. Anything goes. Nothing is valid, and we remain noncommittal. Everything has become interchangeable and unselected. This stands in stark contrast to the Islamist terrorists. We call it diversity, but in its essence it is unselective. We are not in a position to "give birth to stars" as Nietzsche wrote. We cannot defend our narrative and our way of life in a courageous way. We live in a world where "no one wants to die." In contrast, there are young terrorists who are ready to commit suicide while at the same time killing others. There is a nearly unlimited reservoir of young people who are ready for jihad and who are willing to commit terrorist attacks. Two different anthropologies, very different ways of life, and clashing motivations for action.

Sound Judgment and Patience

Terrorists and insurgents are usually rooted in the growing number of failed states and societies undergoing civil war. Some 1.5 billion people currently live in such situations. More than half of the international community of states are classified as fragile. More than 50 million people are refugees. Only a few of them are willing to return to their home countries. To the contrary, those have-nots are desperately seeking shelter in the countries of those who have. Europe has become the "New Jerusalem" for many of these have-nots, since Europe still has rather open borders and is not willing to protect itself appropriately.

With its murderous and brutal hatreds, Daesh is dragging us into counter-reactions. Our resources are tied up. Our hands are knotted. Terrorists want to trigger panic, hatred, insecurity, and retaliation. Their target is to set off a spiral of violence. From their point of view, it is a limitless process, one that will go on and on, since their resources are almost inexhaustible. There will always be someone who is dissatisfied, who feels personally derailed enough to feel dragged into a terrorist network at the right moment. Attacking seems to be a "logical" step.

We shall not please them by allowing them to put our societies in turmoil. Daesh terrorists know well that they are in a no-win situation vis-à-vis Western societies, since we will cut off and destroy their refuges and their infrastructure. Our military and technological capacities and capabilities are far superior to theirs. We are in a position to fight terrorism successfully. For this reason, they must attack our inner social core to break our resistance.

We have to oppose terrorism with sound judgment and patience. In the 1970s, Germany resisted sacrificing fundamental rights and employing unnecessary counterforce when challenged by the radical leftist terror of the RAF. The RAF challenged the German state by trying to "tear off its fascist mask." In addition, Germany avoided reintroduction of the death penalty, although many citizens loudly demanded that the government do so.

As a counterexample, the United States waged a rather senseless war against Iraq. Finally, Iraq descended into total chaos and fell apart. It was and is still definitely worse than ever before. The 9/11 terrorists' calculus proved to be completely successful. They provoked the Western superpower to launch a disproportionate military reaction. Torture was even temporarily legitimized. The secret services were inflated to a new level. Yet, they were powerless to thwart the two "Boston bombers." However, one has to note that there have been no large-scale terrorist attacks on American soil since those broad measures were employed.

Terrorists are usually part-time warriors. They are motivated by idealism and by a number of personal reasons, which are understandable to a certain extent.[6] Many of them try to lift their personal, social, and material status. It is about breaking up the established civil war economy in the countries concerned.

Taking a medium- to long-term stance, a sustainable economic and development policy in the countries concerned will help to counteract the root causes of terrorism. If people have a reasonable and sustainable level of living, fewer will be receptive to radicalism. Educational programs are an additional and important piece of the puzzle in the fight against the root causes of terrorism. It will take huge amounts of money, patience, and time. Such factors as demographic developments, rapid population growth in Africa and the Middle East, little economic prosperity, corruption, weak infrastructure, and conflicts of interest do not provide fertile ground for optimism. Taking demography as a single factor, it does not point in a positive or productive direction. The demography crunch may even force people to join terrorist organizations, since there are virtually no life-affirming alternatives.

Unmanned aerial vehicles (drones) and special forces in the regions of concern are indispensable to minimize the terrorist threat to the free world. Nevertheless, they are highly dangerous if they are not coordinated enough or properly by state authorities, particularly if there is collateral damage among civilians.[7]

Each dead civilian, uninvolved and innocent, is an advertising bonanza for promotion of terrorist activities. In the medium term, education of security forces in these regions may help to influence developments. Eliminating international money flows that are attached to terrorism could constitute a huge asset in countering terrorism. Without money and without logistics, terrorism quickly reaches its limits. Financial support, support in education, technical support, as well as limited military missions and weapons supplies may help to stabilize a region in crisis. Those measures must be accompanied by military means, particularly when it is not possible to act on one's own territory, when police forces are unable to take effective action and armed resistance is simply too strong.

Counterterrorism, stabilization operations, state building, and shoring up key governmental institutions require patience, time, and money. The Balkans, Iraq, and Afghanistan are vivid examples. Another example is the decades-long fight between British security forces and the Irish Republican Army, where there was a high death toll on both sides.

In its essence, it is not about spending more money for our armies, which are not in a position to win wars, as Martin van Creveld rightly highlighted in his book *Pussycat* (2016). It is about a balanced and efficient amalgam of military means, secret service activities, and police-related measures, accompanied by social programs that may constitute the right strategy for countering modern terrorism.

It is about reviving resilience and lost virtues, such as bravery, assertiveness, the will for demographic stability, and clear-cut resistance toward those who want to destroy us. It is about zero tolerance vis-à-vis those who threaten our freedom, the inner core of our societies, in conflict regions and on the global level.

Transnational and Domestic Cooperation

Multilevel cooperation is essential in the fight against terrorism. National egoism has to be overcome, since borders have achieved a different connotation when we talk about global terrorism. Much is communicated via digital media and dark-net channels. Borders have lost their importance on this level of communication. Cooperation must be adapted to these developments.

The connection between cooperation and war has been at the top of the international agenda when talking about fighting terrorism. Particularly since 9/11, the notion of "war" has been regularly injected into the political and societal debate. "War" is a clearly defined notion in international law. Let me offer you some clear remarks. If we want to wage "war" against terrorism, we have already failed and been trapped by the terrorists. Clausewitz defines war as an "extended combat" of at least two opponents. The key goal is to make the opponent defenseless.

Introducing the notion of war in the area of fighting international terrorism automatically implies two opponents who are on the same level, at least in terms of international law. Following this idea, terrorists receive a legitimized position. Western societies deprive themselves of the legal and moral high ground. This concept has to be reconsidered and firmly taken into account when discussing fighting terrorism. Do we want terrorists to be considered on the same level as states? Just think about that!

Another burning issue related to countering terrorism is this: who is better equipped and therefore responsible to fight terrorism? It is generally accepted that the nation-state as a legal construct, and its institutions, which are affected by terrorist attacks, know the operative situation best. They know parallel societies and countercultures, which often are the hotbed for terrorists. For this reason, the nation-state is often much better equipped to undertake appropriate and proportional countermeasures.

National security authorities are usually better off in terms of reconnoitering members of parallel societies. Identifying and fighting them has to be a national chore. However, internationally acting terrorists operate within a number of varieties and groups, thereby leaving national borders outside of consideration. Their modus operandi is transnational in quality and quantity. For this reason, appropriate measures for reasonable cooperation (such as with and between the FBI, Interpol, and Europol) are required to fight terrorism in an efficient and sustainable manner.

Neither our strategic nor our operative course of action must remain only national. Countermeasures must be coordinated and controlled primarily on the state level, thereby integrating state-specific laws and rules. It takes close coordination and cooperation between various secret services, police forces, and law-enforcement authorities located in other states.

Overblown and bureaucratic authorities and unclear competences, particularly in federally organized states such as Germany, constitute the key obstacles for an efficient fight against terrorism. Despite its problematic historic burden, Germany in particular has to accept that it will not be in a position to tackle terrorism without centrally coordinated state-sponsored countermeasures and tight international cooperation between Western secret services and related institutions.

Summing Up

Global terrorism has become one of the most dramatic phenomena during the past 15 years or so. Certainly, some countries are more affected than others, but it is a phenomenon from which no one can detach themselves. It permeates Western societies. For this reason, it is up to those societies to take appropriate measures. The time for talk has passed. Lip service is no longer the right tool. It is time for prudent and strategic action. Some of those actions may be painful. Some may be costly. Some may even curtail our personal freedoms, which have already been diminished by terrorists.

Putting all migrants, returnees, and religiously zealous persons under general suspicion would also play into the hands of the terrorists. It is an important part of their strategy. Activities against the whole group are grist for the mills of their followers who are ready to employ violence. Antiterrorism operations must be finely targeted. Collateral damage has to be avoided at any price. Targeted action requires access to personal data, continuous communication, and an unimpeded exchange of data between secret services and security authorities. Those who do not follow this rule are fetching and promoting terrorism.

It is impossible to wipe out terrorism in a single step with one fatal strike. For the moment, Western societies are forced to live with terrorism. It has become part of our way of life. This does not mean that we accept terrorism as such, but we are trying to understand the phenomenon and its roots and underlying causes, which by itself is most challenging. Yet, it is of utmost importance to come to grips with what is going on and why we are being hit with terrorist attacks so often.

The one who has the stronger will and more endurance will be victorious. At its core, it is an existential fight between two opposing wills, as already described by Clausewitz. It is about making the opponent defenseless. The course of action is highly flexible. It will not follow any fixed rules.

The terrorist's main goal is to act with brute force in a surprising manner at unprotected and unprotectable locations. Creating shock and awe is the meta-goal. The strategy is a long-term project. The number of fighters is uncountable. The reservoir from which to recruit new members is nearly inexhaustible.

Terrorism needs Western societies as a kind of counter-picture, a picture they can hate. It is a mixture of hatred and jealousy, and a deep-seated and often historically burdened feeling of rejection. At the same time, the have-nots desperately try to achieve some standard of living, as many have, by coming to Western societies. It is a parallel picture of "we want at any price" and "we hate for whatever reason."

Sketching the general situation in an overview

- Western societies can be hit anywhere at any time
- The overall vulnerability of societies has been demonstrated
- It is impossible to foresee attacks
- Terrorism creates insecurity among the public
- Public authorities are unable to prevent lone-wolf attacks
- There is a hide-and-seek game going on between terrorists and public authorities

"Action manual" for Western societies

- Regain their core values
- Be mentally and materially prepared for further attacks
- Extend general and particular awareness among the general public that terrorism has become a social phenomenon
- Regain "social media sovereignty"

Patience, prudence, courage, and cooperation are our most important currencies. Cooperation includes micro-/macrolevel collaboration. Since everyone is vulnerable, everyone has to contribute. It is the right mixture that will yield long-term effects in countering terrorism. It has to be complemented by numerous short- and medium-term measures that may include a good deal of self-restriction. This will be a new experience for many of us. It will be a hotbed for a new self-perception of Western societies and what they are capable of doing, particularly in terms of self-affirmation. It is worth thinking about. It is definitely worth doing.

Disclosures

Dr. Erich Vad does not have anything to disclose.

References

1. Elshimi, M. *Thinking about the Symbiotic Relationship between the Media and Terrorism*. Rabat: OCP Center, 2018.

2. Matejic, N. Content wars: Daesh's sophisticated use of communications. *NATO Review*, 2016.

3. National Commission on Terrorist Attacks Upon the United States. *The Financing of the 9/11 Plot*. n.p., n.d.; 2004.

4. Kiger, J. *How Pacifism Works*. History/How Stuff Works, n.p, n.d.; 2016.

5. van Creveld, M. *Pussycats: Why the Rest Keeps Beating the Rest and What Can Be Done about It*. Amazon Digital Service; 2016.

6. Smith, AG. The implicit motives of terrorist groups. *Political Psychology*, 2008; **29**(1): 55–75.

7. Byman, DL. *Why Drones Work: The Case for Washington's Weapon of Choice*. Washington, DC: Brookings; 2013.

Index